YOUR NEW bff

Burn Fat for Fuel

Lose Weight - Beat Diabetes

Kim Minert

YOUR NEW bff

Burn Fat for Fuel

Lose Weight - Beat Diabetes

Kim Minert

INKWELL PRODUCTIONS®

Disclaimer

This material is for informational purposes, and is not intended as a substitute for the advice and care of your physician. Any lifestyle changes should be attempted only after first consulting with your physician to make sure it is appropriate for your individual needs.

The author and her publisher disclaim responsibility for any adverse effects that may result from the use or application of the information contained in this manual.

First printing: February 2016

ISBN: 978-1-939625-34-2

Library of Congress Control Number: 2015912546

Published by Inkwell Productions
10632 North Scottsdale Road, Unit 695
Scottsdale, AZ 85254

Tel. 480-315-3781
E-mail info@inkwellproductions.com
Website www.inkwellproductions.com

Cover photography Dan Watts
Nextworld Media

Printed in the United States of America

Acknowledgement

Giving thanks always and for everything
to God the Father in the name of
our Lord Jesus Christ.
Ephesians 5:20

I would like to thank my husband, Tim, who loves me unconditionally and encouraged me to write as far back as 2002, and has said to me more times than I can remember over the last couple years, "You've got to finish your book!" And did far more than his share of work in the kitchen while I was typing away.

Thank you to my beautiful daughters, Andrea & Alexa, who always support their mom, well, at least put up with her. And for Andrea's contribution writing the exercise chapter of this book and never-ending enthusiasm for going to the gym!

Thank you to my health-conscious parents, Willard and Carole, who are role models in healthy eating and active living, and life-long learners who read books by the hours. They listened, gave feedback, read, edited, and encouraged.

Thank you to my brother, Tim Ferch for writing the recipe section, for his passion for cooking *and* eating delicious food, and for being willing to experiment and convert to low carb cooking. And for not giving up when times are tough, keeping a sense of humor in spite of everything.

Thank you to my BFF, Andrea McNamara for her endless hours listening to me pontificate, rant, and lecture about my newest finds around low carb living. For her contribution of wonderful recipes and low carb holiday meals…and for journeying through life with me.

Thank you to all my *other* BFF's, who are there as a constant encouragement. Whenever I call, you answer! You know who you are. And to my unconditionally accepting friends at Park Central Toastmasters and National Speaker's Association-AZ. No better friends anywhere.

Thank you to my doctor and good friend, Helen Hilts, MD. Founder of *Diabevita*, an educational platform that encourages Low Carb living to prevent diabetes and heart disease. She tirelessly fights the battle on the ground, working one-on-one with her patients and effectively communicating a message of hope that we can all live healthier and happier lives.

And of course, my friend Nick…the founder of Inkwell Productions. He has been both patient and encouraging at the same time. He has helped countless first-time authors like me walk away with a book they can be proud of!

Contributing Authors

Tim Ferch is a foodie and self-taught chef, who made a startling transition to low-carb cooking. His tips and tricks written with humor and tried and true recipes are sure to delight.

Andrea Hall's passion for effective movement is evident in the "exercise" chapter. She writes from the perspective of both personal trainer and ketogenic living expert; you will be inspired and motivated towards healthy living.

Dedication

Randy Glasbergen
Beloved Cartoonist & Illustrator
1957-2015

Randy Glasbergen was a funny guy with a big heart. He struggled like many of us with family history of diabetes, exercise, dieting and managing blood sugar as evidenced by his vast catalog of "toons" on the subject of health. Helping people find joy in the midst of their challenges was a big part of his life. His cartoons make me laugh right out loud.

After seeing one of his cartoons, I found that he had an entire catalog of cartoons on every subject imaginable. We emailed back and forth a couple of times, and I began to pick out my favorites.

When I received the note from his wife, Karen, that Randy had suddenly passed away my heart dropped. She told me that Randy's wish is that she keep his cartoon catalog business running "till the world doesn't need to laugh anymore."

I would like to thank his wife, Karen and his daughter Christie for sharing with me so much about his life, and how many people he helped along the way. After his death, as the cards, letters, and emails began pouring in, they were overwhelmed to hear the heartfelt sentiments of those he had impacted. He not only took a very personal interest in his clients and their needs, he was there to mentor budding cartoonists. Randy published three books for artists desiring to create careers out of their gift for drawing cartoons. He answered inquiries far and wide, no one was too small for him to personally respond to and offer support and encouragement.

Randy began his career as a Professional Cartoonist at age 15, and never stopped. His list of clients include Harvard Business Review, Macy's, Hallmark Cards, International Olympic Committee, IBM, Jeffrey Gitomer, Tony Robbins, Jack Canfield…and many, many more. I am grateful that in the midst of his success, just a few weeks before he passed away, he took the time to answer my email and graciously include the rights to use his cartoons in talks, newsletters and social media.

It is because of his dedication to humanity that I dedicate this book to Randy Glasbergen. Knowing that he ate low carb, exercised, and managed diabetes for the last ten years of his life is a bonus. I know he understood what we are going through… and made us laugh in spite of it. Randy…this book's for you.

Foreward

Why should you read Kim's book? Because it is warm, funny, smart, personal and clear. Eat fat to burn fat and to beat diabetes. Eating low carb/high fat stops the cravings and allows you to lose weight without being hungry. It is simple. The science is well proven and solid. Millions of people have found better health and peaceful weight loss eating this way.

Kim's book is unique because she has experienced all aspects of low carb benefits. She lost weight without being hungry. She kept the weight off without craving. And she easily has much better control of her blood sugars with Type 1 diabetes, the kind that needs insulin from day one.

I was shocked by my own diagnosis of Type 2 diabetes at 48 years old. My first thought was that I would get old fast, fall apart bit by bit and die early. As a physician I knew that our standard treatment of diabetes does not work well and causes cravings. So I studied to find out if a better approach could save me from diabetic doom. What I found was eating low carb prevents and even reverses the complications of diabetes. The science and practical experience are obvious. Now at 60 years old, I still do not need any medicine for diabetes or its comrades, high blood pressure and cholesterol, because of how

I eat. And I lost 26 pounds. In spite of diabetes, Kim and I get to feel good every day.

When Kim first came to my office in 2010, I saw that her blood sugars were "pretty good for a diabetic" but she still experienced damaging highs and dangerous lows. I told her, "We deserve better. We deserve normal blood sugars and long healthy lives, free of struggle with hunger, diabetic complications and constant weight gain."

As Kim says, "My own personal experience created my intense desire to help people with food and diabetes." Practical and down to earth, she explains why and how to switch your fuel from carbs to healthy fats and oils. The book also gives great tools to get past the physical, social and emotional blocks to eating smart and exercising. We really don't have to try and bull through it with will power. You will find yourself thinking, "Oh, I can do this!"

Helen Hilts, MD

TABLE OF CONTENTS

Real Life Success Stories 5
1. What? I'm diabetic? 11
2. The Low Fat Lie 27
3. Insulin & "The Resistance" 35
4. The Diabetes Epidemic 47
5. Are You a Sugar Addict? 57
6. Burning Fat for Fuel 73
7. The Exercise Chapter: The Magic of Muscle 87
8. Making Changes 99
9. Emotional Eating 113
10. Vicki's Story: "I Got My Life Back" 133
11. Eight Obstacles to Low Carb 141
12. What Should I Eat? 151
13. Recipes From The Family Chef... 163
14. Wrapping it all Up 221
Additional Resources 225
Back of the Book 227

INTRODUCTION

In the end, people are persuaded
not by what we say, but by
what they understand.
John C. Maxwell

Just what we need...another book about losing weight. Another eating plan, promising unlimited weight loss while still eating whatever you want. Actually, that's NOT what we need. And that's not what this book is about. This book is for those of us thinking about making a change in eating and life, and who are open to challenging the status quo about what "healthy food" really is. People that carry unwanted pounds or unwanted risks of developing diabetes. Or maybe they have been diagnosed as pre-diabetic or even diabetic. Ouch. It's a book about how a person can make a life-long lifestyle change and never look back, complete with stories of some people who have transitioned and why.

It's for people who lose weight…and then find it again. For people who struggle to get in and out of their cars, and their jeans. Who want to feel good in gym clothes, business clothes, around-the-house clothes, and jammies. People who feel stuck in a job or profession they just tolerate or even despise, because of lack of self-confidence to strike out for what they really want, because of their weight.

And then there's the subject of health. Folks who carry extra pounds are at risk for more health problems than their active healthy friends. Not to say that it's impossible to be a healthy fat guy, it might be. Recent studies show that an active overweight person can be healthier than a thin couch potato. However, if weight is shed, the risk of becoming diabetic goes down drastically! Insulin resistance can be corrected. Hearts don't have to work so hard, nor do knees! Every part of the body will love it.

This book is not just for people who want to lose weight, it is for people who want to be healthy. As a result of the poor nutrition in most of the so-called foods we eat, highly processed foods that are filled with sugar and chemicals, there is a new category of people out there...the skinny fat people. These people may not be visibly suffering, but they are suffering nonetheless and it is going to catch up to them in the form of heart disease and diabetes. It is even more insidious because it is not visibly apparent, and they may not even realize it is happening to them! Scientists are finding that these people, when diagnosed with heart disease or diabetes have a tougher time getting healthy than the guy who needs to lose some weight. A recently published study in the Journal of the American Medical Association reveals the shocking news that nearly 1 in 4 skinny people have pre-diabetes and are "metabolically obese." A new acronym is born. MONW. Metabolically Obese Normal Weight.

America is in the middle of what experts are calling an "Obesity Epidemic." Just over one third of U.S. adults are obese. By the year 2030, it is expected to be 42 percent. Severe obesity will double by 2030, when 11 percent of adults will be nearly 100 pounds overweight.

Trend of obesity among US Adults

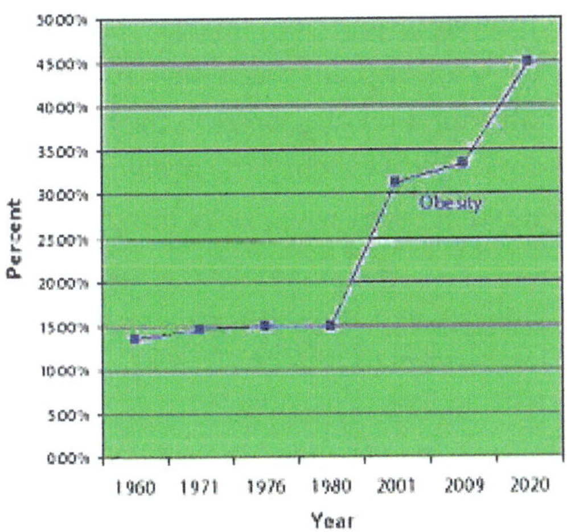

In case you're wondering if this applies to you, obesity is medically defined by having a body mass index of 30 or more. If you are 5'5" and weigh 180 pounds, you are obese. A 5'10" adult hits obesity on the chart at 210. Right here in our country, more than 78 million adults are obese, and sadly, 17% of our children and teens. If you fit the criteria, you are certainly not alone!

According to neuroscientist Sandra Aaodt, it is "dieting's fault." In her Ted Talk she says that we should give people permission to eat whatever they want when they're hungry and stop when they're full. Mindful eating, she says, is "giving yourself permission to eat as much as you want, and then see how your body feels." Then try and use your body's hungry and full feelings to decide how much. She does warn that you will probably not lose weight using this method, and that it took her an entire year to lose her cravings. She also says that doctors don't know of any approach that makes significant weight loss possible for a lot of people, so they are focusing on hoping people do not *gain* weight. The problem is, in her talk, she doesn't tell us what to eat when we're hungry.

And is it really all we can hope for, to stay as fat as we are and never get healthier? I say NO.

Authorities in our country, and many other countries around the world view obesity as one of the most serious public health problems of the 21st Century, and in 2013 the American Medical Association officially classified obesity as a disease. The sad part is that it doesn't have to be this way.

It doesn't have to be this way.

World-wide obesity is a leading preventable cause of death. Prevention is what this book is all about. It is possible to prevent weight gain and obesity, prevent metabolic syndrome and insulin resistance, overcome pre-diabetes, reverse complications of diabetes, and get off drug therapies. We have the power to alter the course of our lives, our health, and our death. There is something we can do win the game, even though we can't change the genetic cards we were dealt. It does, however, require a mindset shift. We have to challenge the wisdom of the day with new information. By eating real food and becoming and staying active we can overcome genetic predispositions, we don't have to get the diseases of our ancestors. We can defy our DNA. Whether you are manifesting symptoms of blood sugar problems at this moment or not, there is no better time than NOW to take action. It's not as hard as you might believe. There is a growing community of support and knowledge surrounding us, let's do it! Defy DNA!

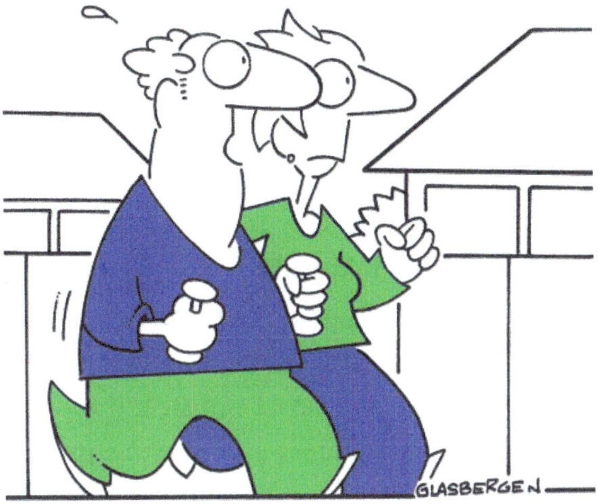

"I blame my weight on bad genetics
I was born with a mouth and a stomach."

STORIES OF REAL PEOPLE

I have struggled for years with a sensitivity to sugar products that would send me down a road of overeating and cravings. I got to a point where I eliminated them from my diet altogether. Then I noticed I craved high carb foods, and the battle was still on. I craved more when I ate them as a steady part of my diet, and there was just never enough to satisfy me. The mental and physical battle dominated.

This summer I had lunch with my longtime friend Kim. After sharing with her the constant battle and struggle of always carrying an extra 20 lbs., and struggling with cravings for chips, popcorn, etc., she explained to me the dynamic of being "insulin resistant" and how it affects blood sugar levels.

My mom was type 2 diabetic, and although I am not diabetic, Kim suggested that I could very possibly be prediabetic. She gave me some reading materials and I went on a low carb eating plan. I have lost 17 lbs. and have not reintroduced high carb foods back into my plan. I have been maintaining my weight and my blood sugars have been steady and the struggle with cravings isn't even there. The craving problem seems non-existent, whereas it had been dominant in my life before.

Could it really be that simple? Kim reassured me that it could be the answer. And it seems to be. Accepting it and learning to eliminate the "high carb" foods on a consistent basis has always been the biggest challenge, but to have my life "settled down" in that way is such a blessing, and it is worth it. Thank you dear friend.

Marilyn Wehmeyer

Kim Minert inspired me to make a lifestyle change that has created wonderful results in two short months. We were talking one morning and somehow the discussion landed on diet and healthy eating. Her eyes lit up and she proceeded to educate me – informing me of how my body responds to carbs and fat and protein – I had heard facts and figures about this type of eating before, but no one had ever given me practical tips and tricks to go low carb. Until then, I had no idea that Kim was an expert in this area – in just a couple of minutes, she clearly explained the basics of how my body metabolizes carbs and fat and I got it, and made some simple changes based on her advice. Now I am 20 pounds lighter, immeasurably healthier and am excited about the prospects for a healthier, happier and much fitter future.

Julie Jennings

"I used to be a super morbidly obese 410-pound man on a one-way ticket to an early grave! After decades of poor eating habits, lack of any meaningful exercise, and just a general apathy about trying to live healthy, it had all caught up to me and I felt trapped thinking this was just the hand I had been dealt with no hope for ever overcoming it. It's a helpless feeling to think you will always be fat and there's nothing you can do about it. And that's EXACTLY what I felt for most of my life."

Jimmy Moore

Jimmy Moore is one of the most prominent bloggers on the low carb lifestyle. At 32 years old, after trying diet after diet, losing and gaining, he found the Atkins diet. It changed his life. In a nutshell, he no longer has to take multiple medications for cholesterol, blood pressure, and breathing problems, and remains over 100 pounds less than his former self! Now at age 43 he maintains robust health while eating low carb.

"Rob was in 5th grade when his grandmother had both her legs amputated."

Rob's story is a great example of meeting the right person at the right time. Sometimes finding the right doctor can be challenging, and when you do find a good one you have to tee it up and be a good patient as well! After a military career spanning 30 plus years, he was required to leave the military medical provision and establish himself with a civilian doctor, using Medicare. At the recommendation of a friend, he made the call to Dr. Helen Hilts in Scottsdale, AZ.

Rob was a foodie from childhood. He not only ate his food, but talked his way into eating his brother and sister's food. He told them it was "yucky" and then when they left it he'd scarf it down! He loved his sweets, cookies, cake, whatever he could get his hands on. Every day was topped off by a dish of ice cream. His transformation "Amazes me!" says his wife, Julie. She said, "Noodles, out of the question. Potatoes, I can't talk him into it! He won't even eat a potato chip!" He's eating low carb, and no alcohol!

You see, Rob was in fifth grade when his grandmother had both her legs amputated, then died just three days later of diabetic complications. He didn't know about diabetes then, or what exactly happened to Grandma. Later as a teenager he found out. When Doctor Hilts told Rob he was pre-diabetic, he said,

"I'm not going to get diabetes, period."

It may have been those traumatic memories that caused him to follow doctor's orders. And follow them he does. And he intends to follow them forever.

Chapter 1

What? I'm Diabetic???

At the age of 44, thin and basically happy with my life, I experienced the shock of a life-time. I have diabetes. The good news… it isn't terminal, it is chronic. Like my dad says, "Chronic means it ain't going away." Diabetes is a chronic disease that must be managed on a daily or even hourly basis, to avoid suffering both long-term and short-term life altering complications. People often ask if I have "the good kind" of diabetes. The fact of the matter is, there is no good kind. The problems created by both Type 1 and Type 2 diabetes are caused by high and low blood sugar levels, and the sad news is that many people don't even know their blood sugar is off kilter until significant damage has occurred.

My own personal experience is a little out of the ordinary, but what happened created my intense desire to help people with food and diabetes. I desperately hope that everyone who knows a diabetic (and who doesn't?) will take the time to learn just a little bit of how life works for us, what doesn't work so well, and take action to stop the dramatic rise of diabetes in our world.

It is my hope that what I've discovered in my journey will help you in yours; you see I live in this mad, mad world every day of my life.

"I live in this mad, mad world of Diabetes every day of my life."

My diabetes was discovered not in a routine doctor appointment, but in a hospital Emergency Room. At the time of my diagnosis I was finally THIN! I had a personal trainer that dragged me out of bed every Saturday morning at 6:00 am. My food portions were similar to what I served my little girls, who were 5 and 8 years old. I hadn't been binging or starving myself like I used to; life was pretty good.

The Christmas Season had passed, and the New Year was upon us. A family tradition, a rousing game of pinochle was what we had planned. I had taught Tim (new boyfriend) to play the game, as it is practically a requirement for those who spend holidays with my family. Mom and Dad were visiting me in Arizona, and Tim was generously hosting New Year's Eve in his little bachelor apartment. He had furnished it with pieces of furniture picked up here and there. We were sitting on wooden chairs with spindles in the back, and I was shifting my body from side to side trying to get comfortable. Tim brought me a pillow to lean against. I had come down with what I thought was a terrible case of the flu just shortly after Christmas. I remember telling Mom. "This flu has really settled into my back!"

We went back to my place, and I tried to sleep, but the fever just wouldn't go away. I rotated Tylenol with Advil, a little trick I used when the girls were babies when their fevers weren't easy to break. But my fever was relentless. 103, 104, 105. It was after one o'clock in the morning and I was burning up. Reaching for the phone on the bedside table, I was barely able to punch the buttons for shaking so much. It took what seemed like an eternity to put in Tim's number. To be honest, I can't even remember what I said to him, but I remember what he said to me. In a worried, almost frantic tone he said, "Go wake up your Mom, right now."

I don't like to be a bother. I am used to taking care of people, not having them take care of me. In spite of my reluctance to wake her up, I dragged myself through the front room to Mom and Dad's door. I told them we had to go to the hospital. I'm sure they were scared to death, not only with worry for their daughter, but wondering how Mom would find the emergency room in a strange city in the middle of the night.

Tim worked his magic on the phone, and guided her right to the door of the emergency room. We managed to park the car and get to the waiting room; me bundled in my sofa blankie. Even though on the surface, the ER didn't seem to be that busy, it took an eternity to see the doctor. I was teetering between burning up and shivering. Finally they brought me back to start the process.

The nurses were awesome that night. They did everything they could to make me comfortable, in spite of a severely crowded emergency department. There were no hospital rooms available.

In triage, they took so much blood it felt like they almost drained me dry. They also performed a weird test to check for the flu, which involved a really long Q-tip and my nose. It was awful. But I was willing to do anything to feel better at that point.

About an hour later, the nurse came back to see me. She wanted to try and squeeze a few more drops of blood out of my arm. She told me, "We think the lab has made a mistake."

Mom and I waited almost the entire night in the emergency room. Finally, the nurse came back in, and asked me point blank, "How have you been managing your diabetes?" Incredulous, I answered, "What diabetes?" She went on to tell me that my blood sugar was 367. Whoa. Normal fasting blood sugar is between 70 and 99, and is not supposed to exceed 140 two hours after a meal. 367 is a very high number.

The nurses were amazed and in disbelief. They had never seen a 44 year old woman who was thin as a rail diagnosed with diabetes. Most people who are diagnosed as adults are generally overweight, have high triglycerides, high cholesterol, and a family history of diabetes. Given that criteria, you would also be Type 2.

I knew quite a bit about diabetes, as I had attended educational classes with, Tim, who is also diabetic. He had been diagnosed with Type 1 diabetes at age 37, again, very rare. I'm sure that God put Tim in my life, He had prepared me with knowledge, and Tim and I would be on this journey together. I knew my high blood sugar reading was an irreversible diagnosis of diabetes. This was a condition I would deal with for the rest of my life. Needles, testing devices, and insulin would be an integral part of my every day existence.

The crowded hospital was unfortunately, a problem for me. Although they made me as comfortable as they could with the intravenous fever reducers and anti-nausea medication, it was a really long night. They told me, "There is no room for you at the inn," and they put me in the pediatric emergency ward. There were a few curtains to prevent me from seeing the crying babies, but I still had to listen to them. There are few sounds more disturbing to a sick, fever infested individual than crying babies. Shrieking is more like it. My mother was incensed that I had to deal with this too, but we had no choice as we waited for the doctor to come pay his "diabetes 101" visit.

Where the scare tactics begin...

The diabetes 101 visit is the scary lecture in which a doctor sounds the alarm to the newly diagnosed diabetic, preparing them to lose their feet, eyesight, and kidney function if they don't keep their blood sugar under control. These are inevitable consequences of non-compliance. According to popular medical opinion it's not a matter if they will happen, but when. And at the time of diagnosis they don't tell you much about how to prevent these things from happening. They send you to a diabetic educator to help you understand the disease and learn how to take care of your new diabetic self. The problem with educators is they usually follow the American Diabetes Association guidelines which tell us to eat too many carbohydrates, making it extremely difficult, if not impossible to manage our disease.

Denial is very easy to do, especially when you are hungry. While we may be concerned about healthy eating overall, we aren't used to evaluating every single bite. Added to that is the problem that most of the health ramifications are not immediate. In addition, we don't look like we have a problem on the outside. That is why diabetes doctors use care tactics upon diagnosis, to try and keep people from denying their disease. Ignoring the situation will result in extreme damage to the blood vessels in the body. The smallest are affected first. Eyes, kidneys, and toes. There's also those little blood vessels in the male sex organ that wreak havoc with mans' reason for living.

To deliver my scare tactic visit, the doctor leaned his back against the one solid wall in my room of curtains. With arms crossed, he began his speech, a speech I'm sure he had given to many people in my situation. But this was not a speech my mom wanted to hear. She was livid. I will never forget the anger on my mom's face as she tried to absorb the words of that doctor.

Now, you'd have to know my mom. She is the sweetest, kindest, most giving person I know. She will drop whatever she is doing to solve someone else's problem. She wouldn't hurt a flea…until she gets mad or someone messes with her children. A mother bear could not be meaner than my mom in the emergency room with a rude doctor trying to scare her baby girl with disastrous consequences of ignoring blood sugar.

Finally, that doctor made his way out of my "room" and the caring nurses returned to let me know they had secured a spot for me upstairs in the hospital. Not in the ward for diabetics, the only available space was in the maternity ward! Moving right up from crying infants to women in labor.

Food Journey after Diabetes Diagnosis

I'll never forget my first meal in the hospital. I had a pork chop, green beans, a biscuit, and some cranberry juice. I asked the young medical assistant if I could have some honey for my biscuit. He looked at the orders and said, "No, you are on a diabetic diet." I started my career in diabetes education right there, trying to teach the kid about nutrition. After all, the second ingredient in the juice drink was high fructose corn syrup. The truth is, a biscuit, beans, corn syrup and honey all have carbs, and they all convert to sugar in your body.

Like a good little soldier who had pretty much been able to control her weight by managing the numbers on the scale and the calories going in her mouth, (talented at being hungry and not eating) I managed to control my blood sugar within the American Diabetes Guidelines. I counted carbohydrates and carefully watched the numbers on my blood sugar monitor. My doctor called me his "poster child" and encouraged me to let people know how I was able to accomplish such good numbers. I thought of my new diabetic self as a car; it was a helpful strategy for me and I also used it to help other people understand my disease. It demonstrates how food and insulin work together.

In choosing a vehicle, there are two basic transmission choices. The manual transmission and the automatic. For most people an automatic is certainly easier to drive. When you want to go faster, you just add fuel by pressing on the gas pedal, and your car automatically and smoothly changes gears to accommodate the needs of the engine.

There is a percentage of the population who prefer to adjust the engine themselves and drive a car with a manual transmission. When the engine begins to race and surge, they get great pleasure out of shoving the clutch to the floor and finding that perfect notch with the gear shift to insure that their transmission will keep up with the new demand of higher speed. A diabetic who learns to drive their disease properly can reach their final destination safely, just like the driver of the manual transmission.

Type 1 diabetics are like the vehicle with the manual transmission. They have to be shifted manually. An insulin injection is the shift that helps the body process the fuel on board. Every bite of carbohydrate must be measured and counted in order for the right gear to be found to keep the engine running smoothly. I used to think I was doing a great job of this, but manually matching insulin doses to fast acting fuel (sugar and starch) perfectly is much more difficult than driving a car with a stick shift, and as I saw by looking at a continuous glucose monitor, nearly impossible.

If the pancreas is healthy and whole, the body perfectly adjusts automatically for increased carbohydrate intake by producing just the right amount of insulin at just the right time to make sure that the blood sugar levels stay at their ideal level.

Diagnosis at age 44 with Type 1 is highly unlikely. So unlikely that most people and even some doctors don't think it can happen, as evidenced by my experience in the emergency room. One time while volunteering at the Phoenix Juvenile Diabetes Research Foundation (JDRF) office, they told me the oldest person they had seen diagnosed was 28. Over 90% of Type 1 cases are diagnosed before the age of 25. Hence the doctor's order to do my blood work over again. I was lucky to have excellent doctors at the onset; they didn't assume that it was Type 2.

The doctor said, "We could try to manage this with pills, but what your body really needs is insulin." It's a big deal, being misdiagnosed is a recipe for disaster in any case. Tim is a good example of a misdiagnosed diabetic. He was 37, and assuming he was Type 2 because of his age, they treated him as such. The first course of treatment for a Type 2 is to give them blood sugar lowering pills, and they gave him Metformin. It is a very good drug according to my doctor, and works by reducing fat in the liver, which in turn allows insulin to work more effectively. However, because his body no longer made insulin, no matter how much he controlled his carbohydrate intake and how much he exercised, he couldn't keep his blood sugar in the normal range. It was two years of struggle before he met a doctor who corrected the diagnosis and treated him properly with insulin.

While diabetes is never good, newly diagnosed adults have an advantage over the kids. The journey of the adolescent diagnosed with diabetes is complicated; teenage emotions, growing pains, puberty. As an adult there is still peer pressure to follow the eating style of the crowd, but as adults we have hopefully gained a sense of perspective, that our health is more important than the pile of pizza on the countertop.

After reading the history of diabetes, I was even more grateful I wasn't diagnosed at an earlier age. The blood glucose monitor was not invented until 1978, and I was a senior in high school. The monitor weighed 3 pounds and was only available in doctor's offices. Diabetics would stand in line to get their blood sugars tested, once a month. Now our monitors are as tiny as a candy bar, weighing in at a few ounces, and we can take them with us everywhere. We can test our blood sugar as often as needed and adjust our blood with insulin or sugar to achieve a number as close as we can to normal.

Upon finding out that I was diabetic, I began doing research. Still dating Tim, he gave me a copy of Dr. Richard Bernstein's book, *The Diabetes Solution*. Dr. Bernstein was diagnosed with Type 1 diabetes at age 12. By the time he was in his thirties, following the standard diabetic care at the time, his body began to deteriorate. He read about the first blood sugar monitor, which was being used in hospitals by emergency room staff to determine if a patient was drunk or had blood sugar problems. Kind of funny that the behavior is similar!

Dr. Bernstein was not a doctor at that time, and he tried to order a monitor. They wouldn't let him have one, because he wasn't a doctor. His wife was, though, and so he had her order it for him. This began his journey to normalize his blood sugar ultimately going on to medical school and devoting his life to helping both diabetics and pre-diabetics normalize their blood sugar. He has written 6 books and at the time of this writing is

81 years old and still working in the clinic he founded near his home in New York. His book has been revised periodically to incorporate the latest findings, adding before and after stories and is, in my opinion, the gold standard for diabetic care.

I'm not sure why I didn't totally embrace his teachings from the very beginning. He is emphatic in his recommendation to drastically lower the carbs and believes eating fat is fine. I wanted to believe that I could keep eating what everyone else around me was eating, and count the carbohydrates. Dose insulin in just the right amount at just the right time and I'm good! As far as my personal diabetes management, I was considered to be exceptional. I did cut back on sugar a little, only eating half a banana or a small piece of desert. Every carefully measured carbohydrate was counted and dosed for. They tell me that my pancreas was still making some insulin, I was in what is known as the honeymoon phase. Blood sugar control was not really a big problem.

But as time moved on and I was still diabetic the next year, and the next, and the next, things became a little more challenging, emotionally as well as physically. There's Thanksgiving, then Christmas. Then Easter, then a birthday dinner for every member of the family. Oh, and those summer barbeques, and Halloween. Did I miss Valentine's Day? New Year's Eve?

Dating a diabetic probably made it a little easier, since we both had to deal with managing blood sugar all the time. People couldn't believe that we both had Type 1 diabetes and were both diagnosed as adults. In fact one doctor said it was like "tossing a coin and having it land on its side." We had been thinking of getting married, and I remember telling Tim, "You have to marry me now, you gave me your disease!"

Even though my averages were good, I knew in secret that I had been experiencing frequent highs and lows, and was starting to get used to seeing a high blood sugar reading of over 200 after a party. Oh well, I'll take my insulin and try to get it down before bed. But it wasn't going down fast enough, and often times I'd go to bed with high numbers. Many times I'd get up in the morning with blood sugars between 160 and 200. My eating habits accounted for a nice average, because I usually didn't eat a large amount of food at a time. I would have a protein shake for breakfast, nibble on a few nuts at lunchtime, and keep the sugars pretty normal during the day. Then I'd eat what is considered a balanced dinner, with a serving of bread or potato or pasta, and most of my after dinner readings would be higher than they should be. Trying to eat carbohydrates and control my sugar with insulin was getting harder and harder.

A good friend mentioned to me that there was a doctor in town who had diabetes herself. Dr. Helen Hilt's number was buried in the notes in my phone, and I dug it up and made an appointment. I went to her website and clicked on a podcast, and an interview she did for a radio program. Her voice was comforting as she described, in the most positive way, "A person can live without carbohydrates, and live well." Like I said, even though I had read *The Diabetes Solution* I still hadn't been able to wrap my head around the idea. I was willing to give up Cinnabons, but all bread, pasta, rice, potatoes forever? It was a stretch for me.

The first appointment was unlike any appointment I had ever had with a doctor. I had asked Tim to join me, since we did, in fact get married. I wanted to share the experience with him and get his buy-in if I was going to undertake a fairly significant lifestyle change. Dr. Hilts introduced herself and began to educate us with her Diabetes 101 for Dummies. She said, "Did you both take science in school? I am going to take this down to basic science."

And basic science is what she showed us. She took out a blue three-ring notebook and flipped from page to page, with drawings of blood cells sticky with sugar. She explained that when blood sugar gets to 160, what I thought was a seemingly harmless number, the blood starts to turn to plastic in your veins. Hmmm, this might explain the damage to those small blood vessels in the eyes, kidneys, feet and other body parts that the doctor in the hospital had warned me about.... She showed us how carbohydrates are just sugar molecules chained together, and have the same potential for destruction as sugar itself. A light bulb went on for me as I remembered what my Mom had been saying about what she was eating.

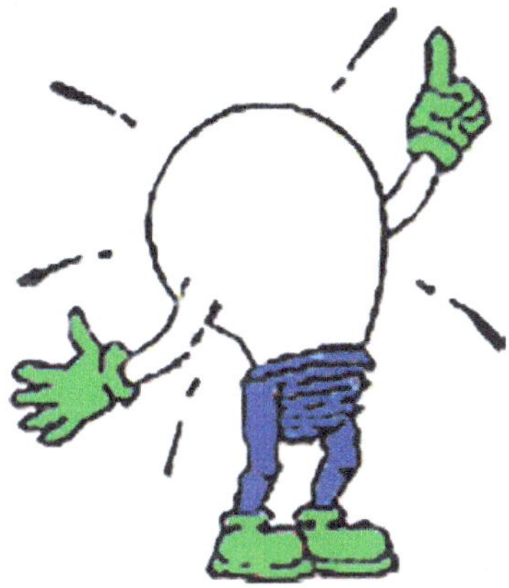

My mother has been a weight loss champion as long as I've known her. It's not that she's followed that many diets to the letter, or that she was even very much overweight. I think it's more like a hobby for her. But after reading the book *"Protein Power,"* by Dr.'s Michael and Mary Dan Eades, she and my dad embraced a low carbohydrate lifestyle. When they first started this new plan, I told them, "You have to have balance! You are not getting the nutrition you need. What about all the fat you're eating?" I hadn't read the book myself, but my conditioning told me they were off target. Dad would try to convince me by telling the story that his friends, "Clen and Barbara went on this diet, and their triglycerides went down, bad cholesterol went down, and good cholesterol went up!" I pooh-poohed the idea; just sure they were in a Protein Power Cult, with Carbohydrates being the devil's scheme. Taking a chomp out of a green pepper was not in the cards for me, and

WHAT? No bun with my burger???

It all came together when Dr. Hilts explained that keeping our diabetes managed by eating low carb is a "beautiful thing." We are not "doomed" as diabetics to live a shorter life filled with complications. With such an optimistic approach how can a girl argue? The beautiful thing is that we can live long, healthy, and productive lives, even with Type 1 diabetes. Type 2 diabetics can reverse their complications, and get off many of the medications that they use to manage their blood sugar. We can all achieve normal blood sugar, and by doing so reduce or eliminate the damage done to our bodies by devastatingly high blood sugar readings on our meters.

CHAPTER 2

The Low Fat Lie

Society at large and the medical community are anchored in the belief that we should eat a low fat diet. That belief is beginning to change slightly, but the dietary community will concede to only "healthy fats". They will allow us nuts, avocado, coconut oil and olive oil…but send daggers of fear into our hearts if we eat saturated fat.

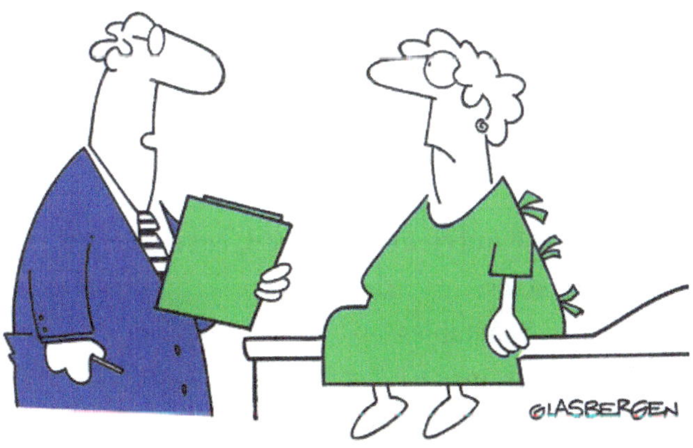

"The high-carb diet I put you on 20 years ago gave you diabetes, high blood pressure, and heart disease. Oops."

The following misinformation comes directly from the American Heart Association. **Do not believe most of the following…**

"Saturated fats occur naturally in many foods. (True) The majority come mainly from animal sources, including meat and dairy products. (Also true)

Examples are:

- fatty beef
- lamb
- pork
- poultry with skin
- beef fat (tallow)
- lard and cream
- butter
- cheese
- other dairy products made from whole or reduced-fat (2 percent) milk.

In addition, many baked goods and fried foods can contain high levels of saturated fats.

To get the nutrients you need, eat a dietary pattern that emphasizes:

- fruits, vegetables
- whole grains
- low-fat dairy products
- poultry, fish and nuts
- less red meat, sugary foods and beverages

Choose lean meats and poultry without skin and prepare them without added saturated and Trans fats.

You should replace foods high in saturated fats with foods high in monounsaturated and/or polyunsaturated fats. This means eating foods made with liquid vegetable oil but not tropical oils. It also means eating fish and nuts. You also might try to replace some of the meat you eat with beans or legumes.

Four Things that are Wrong with this Story.

1. Fruits are what Dr. Andreas Eenfeldt calls, "nature's candy." They should not be first on the list, and with the exception of berries which have less sugar and more fiber, should be eaten sparingly if at all.
2. Vegetables should exclude starchy vegetables, corn and potatoes being the top two carby culprits. Dr. Ron Rosedale calls a potato a "lump of sugar."
3. Whole grains turn to sugar, starting in your mouth as you chew them.
4. The high fat foods that keep you full are barely allowed, therefore guaranteeing you will be hungry most of the time.

It is urgent that we learn the truth about dietary fat. Not only is eating fat not evil, it is in fact necessary. Dr. Steven Phinney, a leading doctor in the field, coined the word *keto-adaptation* in

1980. Our bodies can adapt to burning fat for fuel and thereby create a steady stream of energy… and it's much more efficient than fast-burning carbohydrates.

Expert's Answers aren't Solutions

Many of the so called experts in the medical field offer dietary answers that research shows are not solutions to the problems of obesity and diabetes. For example, Harvard Health Publication writers say, "Emphasize complex carbohydrates, fruits, vegetables, whole grains, and lean protein." We all agree that "bad food" includes white bread, refined-grain pasta, and sugary drinks, but only eliminating the "white" version of those carbohydrate-laden foods and sugar-filled beverages will not solve the problem.

A lot of Americans have already switched from white bread to whole wheat, from white rice to brown. From regular pasta to whole wheat pasta, and from white potatoes to sweet potatoes. Some people have heard about the glycemic index, which classifies food relative to how fast it raises your blood sugar. They then try to eat carbohydrates that are low on the glycemic scale. The glycemic scale measures the effect of a food on blood sugar comparing it to pure glucose. If the scale classifies a carb as low glycemic, it means it raises your blood sugar slower than glucose, but the key word here is raises. That's right, folks, the darn blood sugar still goes up! That is why eating whole grains doesn't solve the problem.

How did we arrive at this place, filling our bodies with empty carbohydrates that cause hunger, while declaring fat the enemy and taking it out of our foods, even though it keeps us full? Let's take a look at the history of the low fat movement; it's clear to see how we got here.

History of Low Fat Ideology

1862: Establishment of the United States Department of Agriculture (USDA).
Its two main objectives were to make sure we had enough food to sustain our citizens and to provide information on subjects related to agriculture.

1917: USDA laid out five basic food groups.

1. Fruits and Vegetables
2. Meats and other Protein Foods
3. Cereals and other Starchy Foods
4. Sweets
5. Fatty Foods

1958: The five groups were reduced to four.

1. Milk
2. Meat
3. Vegetable/Fruit
4. Bread/Cereal

1968: The Senate appointed George McGovern chairman of the Select Committee on Nutrition and Human Needs.
This bipartisan committee met until 1977 when they

issued this report:

1977: Americans need to eat more fruits, vegetables, whole grains, poultry, and fish, less meat, eggs, and high-fat foods, and they should substitute non-fat for whole milk.
This report, also referred to as the "McGovern Report," first used the term *complex carbohydrate*, denoting "fruit, vegetables, and whole-grains." The federal government officially supported the high carbohydrate low fat approach and in 1978-79 the American Society of Clinical Nutritionists and the National Cancer Institute recommended a diet low in fat as well.

1980: A scientific consensus was emerging that a low fat diet was needed to prevent heart disease and cancer. By the end of the decade, in spite of protests from the food industry and skeptical scientists, both the Surgeon General's Report on Nutrition and Health and the World Health Organization were promoting low fat.

1988: American Heart Association issued its "heart healthy" seal of approval. Food companies paid money to label their foods with the seal of approval. By 1990 these food products appeared in grocery stores. (Fresh foods were not labeled)

1992: The food pyramid supported the ideology of low-fat.
1997: Fifty-five companies had the heart healthy seal with over 600 products certified, including Frosted Flakes, Fruity Marshmallow Krispies, and Low Fat Pop Tarts.

Now you can see how low fat high sugar products were being perceived as "healthy". It was possible to believe that if a product was low in fat, you could eat as much as you wanted! We have been sold a bill of goods. The numbers don't add up. A lot of my friends who have been living low fat, eating oatmeal with skim milk and salads with low fat dressing, are struggling. Some are accumulating unwanted fat around their mid-section, and many often ask me what I am eating, how much I exercise, and how I keep my girlish figure. Ha! That is a major reason I am writing this book now. I hope to communicate what has worked for me and what is working for many other people. It can work for you.

CHAPTER 3

Insulin & "The Resistance"

Insulin is a naturally occurring hormone produced by beta cells located in the pancreas. Its job is to regulate the flow of energy throughout the body, and keep our blood sugar within the normal range. Day and night, your pancreas releases insulin depending on your needs. The sugar in our blood gives us energy, and the insulin is a gatekeeper, opening the gate to the cell and allowing our bodies to use glucose for energy. This is a very good thing. But if we eat more than we can effectively use, insulin becomes a very efficient fat-storing agent, storing fat in the cells most receptive to holding it. It saves it for hard times, when food isn't as easy to get. Like during the depression in the 1930's. The problem is that we haven't had a food dry-spell for a long time but we keep storing up, just in case!

Another one of insulin's main functions is to shut down fat release following a meal, according to obesity researcher Stephan Guyenet, Ph.D. of the University of Washington. Wow. I don't want too much of that going on!

1. **Insulin lets glucose into the cell**
2. **Insulin stores fat**
3. **Insulin stops fat release after a meal**

Sometimes more of a good thing is not always better, and that is the case with insulin. In the right amounts, insulin is vital to life itself. If we did not make any, we would die. If I would have been diagnosed with diabetes before insulin was discovered in 1921 for use in humans (they tried it out on dogs at first), I would have had only a few weeks or months to live, and maybe up to a year if I ate almost nothing. Before 1921, that was the only treatment option available. Diabetics were instructed to basically stop eating.

My great aunt, my grandma's sister, Myrtle Sorenson, had Type 1 diabetes, and is the only family member I know of with Type 1 except me. She was born in 1919 in rural Wisconsin, and I have no way of knowing when she developed diabetes or when she was diagnosed. I was told that she did have insulin at some point, but she apparently would sneak off when her mother wasn't looking and eat candy. Sadly she slipped into a diabetic coma and died at the age of 13. You can understand my motivation to keep injecting myself with insulin. Shots? Not a problem given the options. This is what Tom Nikkola, co-owner of Healthy Living How To says about insulin.

"The most significant factor in fat storage is the level of insulin in the blood. Insulin has many effects on the body. With respect to fat storage, insulin increases the storage of fat in fat cells and prevents fat cells from releasing fat for energy."

"Insulin increases the storage of fat in fat cells and prevents the cells from releasing fat for energy."

In his bestselling book, *Good Calories, Bad Calories*, Gary Taubes has this to say, "Refined carbohydrates raise your insulin levels. Scientists have known since the early 1960s that insulin is the primary hormone that regulates your fat tissue. This is not controversial—if you go and find an endocrinology textbook and look up what makes a fat cell fat, it'll tell you all the ways insulin does it. Then you look up obesity, and it'll say people get fat because they eat too much and exercise too little. There's a complete disconnect between fundamental science and the cause of human obesity."

"There's a complete disconnect between fundamental science and the cause of human obesity."
Gary Taubes

Insulin resistance is a condition in which the gates to our cells are difficult to open, and consequently the cells can't get the energy they need for fuel. It is a very unfortunate state. It is the driver behind cravings and fat storage. Insulin resistance is also the common denominator for people with hypoglycemia. This is how it works. The pancreas releases insulin, starting when we taste something sweet and ideally makes just the right amount to cope with the carbohydrate count. The insulin unlocks the gate and tells the muscle, liver and fat cells to use the glucose provided by the carbs for energy. Hopefully all the glucose and insulin are used up, because if there is too much sugar or insulin in the blood it is toxic for the body. Because of this toxicity, our bodies try, at all costs, to keep blood sugar normal! So the beta cells in the pancreas sense insulin resistance, and shove out too much insulin. Because of this extra production, there is more than enough insulin in the blood, which stores more fat. To give you a real-life example, if you eat one chocolate chip cookie, your body makes enough insulin for four to ten cookies. After you eat the one cookie, your insulin level gets too high and then plummets. This drop in blood sugar causes the symptoms of hypoglycemia, shaky hungry feelings, and when you eat carbohydrates again the cycle repeats.

Given the high levels of insulin, the body is in a perfect state to store fat, just in case you need extra energy in times of famine. Or hibernation, as in the case of the mother bear. In the fall, berries are plentiful and by God's design the bear becomes insulin resistant. She eats and eats, storing plenty of fat to get her through the winter. This insulin resistance works great for the bear, but not so much for humans who never hibernate.

Our insulin resistance and easy access to carbohydrate-laden food have created a perfect environment for us to develop diabetes. It looks something like this:

We get up in the morning, eat a bowl of cereal and a banana. The cereal turns to sugar in our mouths within seconds of being hit with saliva. If you don't believe me, Dr. Richard Bernstein, in his book, *Diabetes Solution* says you can see if what you are eating turns to sugar if you hold it in your mouth for just a few seconds and spit on a ketone stick. When the color changes you can see which foods converts to sugar. Okay, back to breakfast. The cereal turns to sugar (all grains do) and the milk has sugar (lactose) and so does the banana (fructose). BAM. Sugar overload. This food doesn't keep energy levels stable or keep us full till lunch, so a mid-morning snack is in order. It might be a muffin. Go to www.sugarstacks.com and you will find that a very healthy-looking bran muffin from Starbucks topples about 6 teaspoons of sugar into your bloodstream. You feel a little better though, and manage to make it to lunch.

Wanting to lose a few pounds, you order a "salad" for lunch. Salad can be a carbohydrate loaded meal or something moderately healthy. If it has grapes, mandarin oranges, raisins, or apples it is loaded with sugar before they add the poppy seed dressing! Maybe your salad has a few bites of chicken, you feel good about it because it's the breast. You know, low fat. This meal won't keep you full for long, and in my experience I'm hungry for a snack by 4:00 in the afternoon. Cookies in the break room…or ANYTHING. I'm hungry.

Somehow we make it to dinner, and thankfully have a substantial serving of protein. And a vegetable. Feeling pretty good about our food day. Until we decide to have desert before bed! Or popcorn. Yummmm.

This type of eating causes beta cells to produce a boatload of insulin starting with breakfast, even though we didn't technically overeat or binge, and felt like it was a pretty good food day. Those beta cells got the workout of their lives. Think about those overworked cells as a friend you love and care about. You would want your friend to take a break, rest, and refresh. Without that much needed rest, burnout is the predictable outcome.

The only way to rest your beta cells, thereby extending their lives, is to eat less carbohydrates. By eliminating the root cause of excessive insulin production, you give your beta cells a fighting chance. I know you can do it!

> *When a doctor says his patient has insulin resistance, he does little to enlighten the patient. Rather, the term insulin resistance creates a sense of mystery. On the other hand, when we say the cell membranes are toxic and plasticized, rendering immobile the insulin receptor embedded in them, we sharply define what the problem is: hardened and dysfunctional cell membranes.*
>
> *Majid Ale*

As a Type 1 diabetic I don't make insulin at all. ANY carbohydrate, complex or not, RAISES MY BLOOD SUGAR and requires insulin. It doesn't make any difference where the food falls on the glycemic scale.

Whole wheat bread isn't better than white… a carb is a carb, the numbers don't lie. Take a good look at the carbohydrate count on a package of whole grain pasta! It is frightening that so-called experts are telling us that eating whole grains is part of the answer. Their answers are not solutions.

Their Answers are Not Solutions

Every day of the week poor unsuspecting patients go to the doctor and are told to eat whole grains and less fat and exercise more. How many times have they tried it and failed? So many times. And obesity is on the rise and along with it diabetes and other related diseases.

Scientists are hoping to develop a drug treatment to cure us from storing abdominal fat. Now there's a cool idea! Pop a pill and solve the problem. Hasn't happened yet, unfortunately, so here's what we're left with, "Experts think for now the best way to fight fat is in the way we live our lives." Finally the experts have something right. Now if they would just embrace the lifestyle that really solves the problem.

How We Become Diabetic

In a healthy body every part is working properly. The pancreas doesn't have to work too hard to process a moderate intake of carbohydrates, the muscles, liver, and fat cells have room to store the glucose, and the person is pretty happy with consistent energy and normal weight.

If that person develops insulin resistance, eats too many carbohydrates for his personal tolerance, he is not able to keep the sugar levels within a normal range. A fasting glucose tolerance test is what determines the level of sugar in the blood. When a doctor announces a fasting blood sugar of 90, it is a sure sign of insulin resistance. When it goes above 99, physicians will wave a warning flag of pre-diabetes. If fasting blood sugar hits 126, it's a diagnosis of diabetes.

Sadly, most people don't get the education and support they need in the early stages,that could delay or even prevent the actual diagnosis. People think, "I'm just pre-diabetic." Nobody tells them that in the pre-diabetic stage, half of their insulin producing beta cells are already used up. We have all the beta cells we will ever have by the age of five, and they are supposed to last a lifetime. In order for them to keep producing insulin for as long as possible, the best thing to do at this point is rest the remaining cells.

Insulin resistance shows up, overworking the cells, long before weight gain or symptoms like excessive thirst. In light of this information, it is extremely important that all of us ask our doctors to test for insulin resistance and high blood sugar.

Researchers and scientists have been sounding the alarm since the early 2000's, and it's time we all pay attention. The problem is an imbalance of carbohydrate/fat/protein in our diets, and the answer is found in whole natural food itself, with the majority of calories coming from, I know, hard to believe... fat. Fat, unlike carbohydrates and part of our protein intake, does not trigger an insulin response, and provides steady fuel. Dr. Eric Westman reminds us constantly, "Eat fat to burn fat". Just to be clear, what he means is when you eat fat and restrict carbohydrates, your body will burn the fat you eat and also the body fat that's already been stored. If we truly want to burn stored fat, we have to overcome the fear of eating fat and reject the low fat message that we have been spoon fed for years.

When fat shows up around the waistline, it is a sure sign of "The Resistance." Most people think that gaining weight causes insulin resistance, but some leading physicians and researchers are pointing to the reverse, that it is the resistance that accelerates fat storing. It is a cycle that needs to be broken in order to regain our svelte physiques and good health! Current studies even indicate that the fat we have stored is biologically active, producing hormones that affect our heath. Whoa! Harvard Health Publications (February 2007) even goes so far as to say that you can think of fat as an endocrine organ or gland.

What exactly does this mean? Well, when we have fat around our middle we just think it's a sign that we regularly eat more than we should. But it seems there's more to it than that. Scientists are still trying to figure it all out, but through research it is becoming clear that too much fat stored on our bodies disrupts the normal balance and function of our hormones. This evil body fat pumps out chemicals that creates even more insulin resistance, diabetes, heart disease, high blood pressure and poor blood clotting. It is also, without question, directly linked to higher total cholesterol and bad cholesterol, and lower good cholesterol. Studies are not only being carried out in the United States, but around the world.

Anja Rosenow, leading researcher at Maastricht University, Department of Human Biology in the Netherlands and her colleagues report on this hormone producing activity, and have found that one of the hormones produced is leptin, which controls appetite, and adiponectin, which works with insulin sensitivity and blood sugar levels.

To see if you are at risk for insulin resistance, measure your waist and hips. A man who has a waist bigger than his hips and a woman whose waist is 80% as big around as her hips, should be on the alert. Using these guidelines, if your waist measurements are within the range, Dr. Richard Bernstein says you are "viscerally obese". The viscera are the intestines and visceral fat is stored within the abdomen and surrounds a number of important internal organs such as the liver, pancreas and intestines. This makes this kind of fat more dangerous than subcutaneous fat, which is just under the skin. Dr. Bernstein also adds "the ones that eventually become diabetic are the ones that can't make enough insulin to keep up with their intake of carbohydrate."

Gary Scheiner, Certified Diabetes Educator and author of the book, *Think like a Pancreas,* uses a great word picture of insulin resistance and the progression of Type 2 diabetes. Let's say you are running an air conditioner to keep your house a certain temperature in the summer. When it warms up outside, the air conditioner kicks on as needed to keep the house temperature "normal." But what if your system has a leak and blows cool air instead of cold? The unit would run most of the time, and eventually wear out. Just like a machine will run for its estimated hours of usage, so the insulin producing beta cells in our pancreas have a limited amount of time to keep our bodies running like a finely tuned engine. As the pancreas begins to burn out, the production of insulin can no longer keep up, and BAM. You're diabetic.

CHAPTER 4

The Diabetes Epidemic

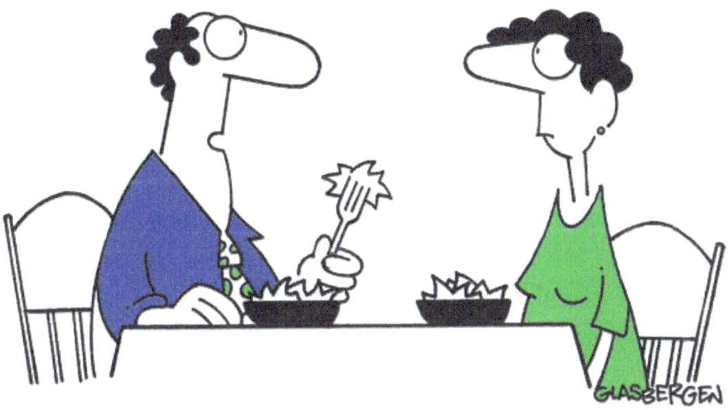

"My doctor says I'm a Type 8 diabetic...that's a Type 2 with four times more excuses for not exercising."

One of the first questions people ask me whenever the subject of diabetes comes up, is the difference between Type 1 (formerly Juvenile Diabetes) and Type 2 (formerly called Adult Onset Diabetes).

Type 1 is an autoimmune disease. It has a genetic component, but is not necessarily considered to be hereditary. It is thought to be triggered by a virus, and the body attacks itself and kills off the insulin producing beta cells located in the pancreas. Ten percent of diabetics are Type 1, and only ten percent are diagnosed as adults.

Type 2 comes into play when the body can't make enough insulin to keep up with the carb load, and blood sugars rise. It is usually genetic. If you are overweight, particularly if you carry weight around the middle, over 45, have a family history, been diagnosed with fatty liver or gout, or are Black, Hispanic, American Indian, or Asian American, or have an inactive lifestyle you have a higher risk of developing Type 2. It is important to know the risk factors and talk to your doctor of you suspect you may be on the road to diabetes.

Seven Risk Factors for Diabetes

1. **Weight gain at the waistline**
2. **Over 45 years old**
3. **Have a family history of diabetes**
4. **Have fatty liver**
5. **Have gout**
6. **Are Black, Asian-American, Hispanic, or American Indian**
7. **Have an inactive lifestyle**

Many Americans do not know they are at risk, they could have insulin resistance, they could be pre-diabetic or even have diabetes and don't even know it. If they do, they might not know what to do about it. The United States Center for Disease Control, in its 2014 report, estimates that there are 8.1 million people with diabetes who are undiagnosed, which is 27.8% of all diabetics. This is extremely disturbing, because of the many diseases people develop in their life-times, diabetes is one disease over which we have a lot of control.

> *"Though no one can go back and make a brand new start, anyone can start now and make a brand new ending."*
>
> *Carl Bard*

I do not want to believe, even in the face of daunting evidence and statistics, that you or I have to develop insulin resistance, get fat, and progress to a diagnosis of diabetes. That we are doomed to be overweight or unhealthy, and if we go on a diet and lose weight we're probably going to gain back anyway.

I don't want to believe it, but the fact is most of us DO gain it back, and 5 years after losing the weight 40% have even gained more. These statistics could make even the most optimistic in our ranks lose heart!

We need a much more strategic plan than the "eat low fat, eat whole grains, exercise more" strategy, because following this plan we lose some weight and then turn right around and find it again.

As a society we are hopelessly addicted to carbohydrates, hungry from eating low fat, and the addiction fights us every step of the way until we are fat again and even fatter than before. This is depressing, sad, and so very costly.

Huge dollars are spent on healthcare for obesity, and much, much more for diabetics. The American Diabetes Association claims that the total estimated cost of diagnosed diabetes in 2012 was $245 billion, including $176 billion in direct medical costs and $69 billion in reduced productivity.

People with diagnosed diabetes spend about $13,700 per year on medical treatment, of which about $7,900 is attributed to diabetes. These folks spend an average of 2.3 times more in medical costs than people without diabetes.

According to Dr. Robert Lustig, UCSF Professor of Pediatrics in the Division of Endocrinology, in his book *Fat Chance, the Hidden Truth about Sugar* writes, "We have to do something about it, or there will be no healthcare. In fact, there will be no society. Are you ready for that? That's what's gonna happen. It's just not OK. There will be no money left for anything else."

Diabetes causes 10,000 new cases of blindness in the US every year. 44% of new cases of kidney failure in 2011 were attributed to diabetes. Over 2 million people of all ages with kidney failure are living on dialysis or had a kidney transplant because of diabetes. 60% of non-trauma foot and leg amputations in people over the age of 20 occur in people with diabetes.

This is a dire situation. A National Emergency. Our kids are getting fatter, and Type 2 diabetes is creeping down to the youngest of our children. 5, 6, and 7 year olds are being diagnosed! A child from Houston, Texas is the youngest ever, her parents brought her to the doctor at the age of 3. She was diagnosed because of the typical signs of diabetes. She had gained a lot of weight, was very thirsty, and had to go the bathroom more than normal. She was in the heaviest 5% of children her age. Doctors put her on metformin, an oral medicine for Type 2 diabetes, and her parents got on board with diet and exercise. The good news…hers was a huge success story at the European Conference on Diabetes in Stockholm, Sweden for reversing all her diabetic symptoms. Within six months she lost 75% of her weight and normalized her blood sugar. It can be done!

According to Francine Ratner Kaufman, MD and many other experts, the most significant risk factor for diabetes is obesity. She tells us that 15-20% of America's teens are overweight. This amounts to more than 5 million children at risk for diabetes.

And there's the "skinny fat kid". Dr. Mark Hyman, author of *The Blood Sugar Solution,* who has dedicated himself to researching the root of the problem reports, "Studies on teenagers found that 37% of the skinny kids had one or more signs of pre-diabetes such as high blood pressure, high blood sugar, or high cholesterol." Wait – almost 4 out of 10 of normal weight kids are pre-diabetic?

Understanding the financial costs to ourselves and to our healthcare system is one thing. But what about the costs to ourselves as human beings? I've heard the devastation in the voices of newly diagnosed diabetics, and the frustration of those who are struggling to control it. They've done everything right, according to the guidelines set by the American Diabetes Association and endorsed by our government. They may have read countless books about diabetes, with conflicting messages which cause even more confusion. Following these guidelines their blood glucose numbers might get a little bit better, but not even close to normal healthy levels.

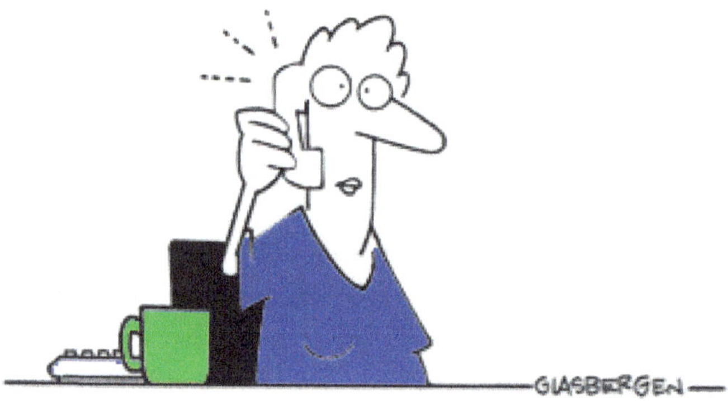

"Welcome to the Diabetic Hotline! If you need a new excuse for cheating on your diet, press 1. If you need a new excuse for skipping your workout, press 2...."

Education is part of the equation, for sure. Hopefully the medical community will embrace the truth that we can prevent diabetes, and begin to educate their patients. Hopefully patients will hear the good news from the whistle blowers, become early adopters, and ask their physicians for better care. They'll learn that they deserve to have a vibrant life with energy to spare.

What does Normal Blood Sugar have to do with it?

While it is a wonderful thing to set ourselves free from letting numbers on the scale determine our self-worth, if you are pre-diabetic or diabetic, there are some numbers that really do matter for long term health…and short term too, as far as that goes.

A tragic, but fairly frequent, thing that happens to Type 1 diabetic young people is when they drink alcohol they often don't eat. When their blood sugar drops, they feel drunk, and their friends assume they are drunk. When they pass out, same thing. Friends don't realize they have a serious problem, they slip into a diabetic coma and it is sometimes too late; they die. Of course this could happen to older people as well.

On the flip side, high blood sugars are damaging in the long term. In the case of Type 2, sugar levels increase gradually over time, their body adjusts to it, so they feel fine. That is the subtle scheme of diabetes. Compare it to rust. Slow oxidation over time turns the underside of your car to a brown powdery substance, and high blood sugars over time turn your blood into a brown gooey substance. Blood in this state can't circulate freely and provide your body the nutrients it needs. This is one major commonality between Type 1 and Type 2, the risk of running high blood sugar.

Alc	Avbs*		Alc	Avbs*	
4.5	83	Optimal	6.5	154	Diabetes
4.6	83		6.6	158	
4.7	90	Sub-Optimal	6.7	161	
4.8	93		6.8	165	
4.9	97		6.9	168	
5.0	101		7.0	172	
5.1	104		7.1	176	Harmful
5.2	108	Normal	7.2	180	
5.3	111		7.3	183	
5.4	115		7.4	186	
5.5	118		7.5	190	
5.6	122		7.6	193	
5.7	126	Pre-Diabetes	7.7	197	
5.8	129		7.8	200	
5.9	133		7.9	204	
6.0	136		8.0	207	
6.1	140		8.5	225	Dangerous
6.2	143		9.0	243	
6.3	147		9.5	261	
6.4	151		10.0	279	

* average blood sugar

One of the essential numbers in the life of a diabetic is the "quarterly report" number that we get when we have blood work done every three months. It is called the "Hemoglobin A1c," and it measures the amount of glucose on each little red blood cell. The amount of sugar on the cell gives us an accurate picture of how our blood sugars have been doing over a three month period. You can run, but you cannot hide.

You can use the numbers on the chart either way. If you track your blood sugar on a regular basis you can correlate your average and get a good idea of what your A1c number will be when you see your doctor. Once your doctor has given you the A1c number, you can see what your averages have been.

The American Diabetes Association recommends that a number of 7 is a target A1c for most diabetics. However, if you look at a 7 on this chart you will see that it correlates with an average blood sugar of 172. Since normal non-diabetic blood sugar is 80-120, I don't think I want to have an average of 172.

Dr. Helen Hilts told me that if my blood sugar gets to 160 it will have the same chemical action as in making plastic. People lose their toes, feet, and legs because of blood plasticising in their veins, even the cell structure is affected. A scare tactic for sure, but you can't argue with science.

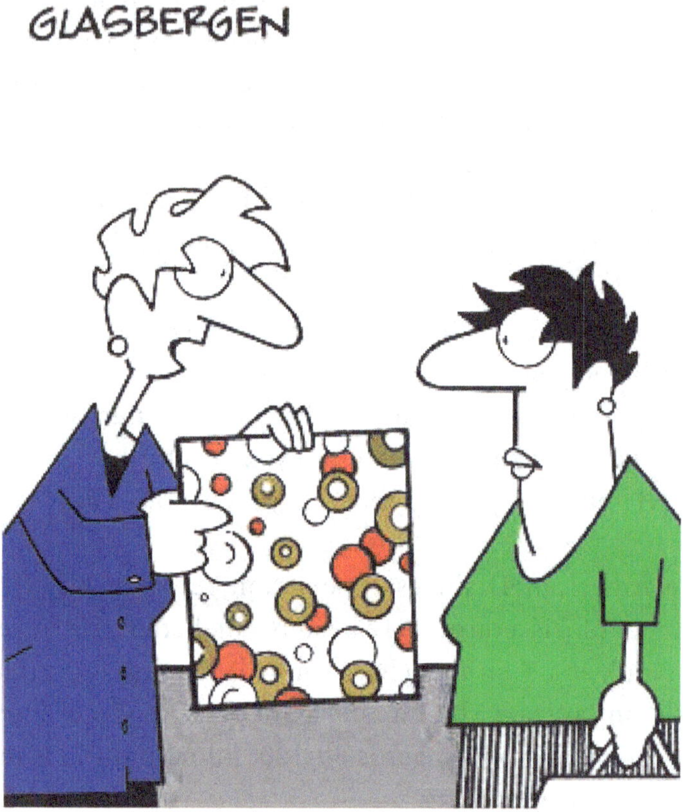

"The red circles are your red blood cells.
The white circles are your white blood cells.
The brown circles are donuts. We need to talk."

CHAPTER 5

Are You a Sugar Addict?

When researching sugar, I found that sugar is more complicated than I thought! For the purposes of this book, I want to explore just the surface, to create a basis for understanding of how it works in our bodies.

Sugar is a single molecule carbohydrate, a molecule consisting of Carbon, Oxygen, and Hydrogen. Hence the name…Carb O Hydrate. A starch is a complex carbohydrate, which is simply a chain of sugar molecules strung together. Amylase is an enzyme, found in our saliva and in our intestines, which breaks the starch (chains of sugar) into simple sugars, like glucose, fructose, and sucrose.

Glucose is also called blood sugar, as glucose is what circulates in the blood. The body breaks down most carbohydrates we eat into glucose, and it's used for energy or is stored as fat in muscle cells or the liver.

Fructose is found in fruits and vegetables, and is added to

many of our foods and beverages. It is processed differently in our body, and is not our body's favorite when it comes an energy source. It is only metabolized in the liver, and is more fat-producing than glucose. Because of this, we now know of the danger of extremely high intake of fructose. Even the media is talking about the need for a reduction of it in our diets. The use of high fructose peaked in the 1990s and is tapering off, because the public became aware of the connection to obesity and diabetes and demanded changes.

Sucrose is made from sugar cane or sugar beets and also occurs naturally in fruits and vegetables. When we eat it, our body separates it into individual units of glucose and fructose. We respond to the glucose and fructose by making insulin, and any extra energy that is not immediately used is stored as fat; stimulated by the insulin released. In fact, it may be hard to believe, but anything that even *tastes* sweet causes us to release insulin.

According to pediatric endocrinologist Dr. Robert Lustig, when we eat foods that contain a lot of sugar, our brain releases a massive amount of dopamine. Eating them often, and in large amounts, causes the dopamine receptors to decrease. With fewer receptors, their effect is lessened and we need more and more sugar to feel as good as we did the last time we ate it. Dr. Lustig adds that sugar, because of its power to affect the reward centers of the brain, works in a similar manner as drugs of abuse like cocaine and nicotine.

In a study published in NeuroImage Magazine, researchers used MRI's to test which areas of the brain are involved when we consume sugar. It is no surprise that all three parts of the brain, hippocampus, caudate, and insula are identical in both food cravings and drug addiction. We definitely don't have a need for cocaine or nicotine. If it were true that our cravings indicate our bodies' needs, we would have overwhelming urges to eat spinach and Brussels sprouts!

QUIZ: Are you a Sugar Addict?

Answer yes or no to the following:

1. If you reach for one cookie or chip, is the bag empty before you know it?

2. Can you skip dessert but empty the bread basket — and the pasta platter?

3. Can you control your food intake during meals but lose it when you start to snack, especially on chips and crackers?

4. When you want to lose weight, is it easier to skip meals altogether rather than eat smaller ones?

5. Are you tired all the time? Are there things you'd love to do but just don't have the energy for?

6. Once you've had "just a taste" of bread, bagels, muffins, crackers, pasta, or rice, do you go back for a second (or third) helping?

7. Do you spend the day on a roller coaster of snacking highs and lows, hitting the doughnuts in the morning, the vending machine chips or candy in the afternoon, and the ice cream at night?

8. Do you eat healthy around other people but lose it when you're alone?

- If you answered yes to two or more odd-numbered questions, you are probably addicted to sweets or salty snacks—cookies, chips, cakes—that have been carefully engineered by food scientists to keep you eating and eating and eating.
- If you answered yes to two or more even-numbered questions, you are highly susceptible to the addictive powers of white flour (which acts like sugar during digestion).
- If you answered yes to two or more odd- and even-numbered questions (at least four total questions), you are highly susceptible to food addiction, period.

There is a way out and education is your first line of defense.

Knowing about the addictive nature of sugar lets you off the hook, even if just a little bit. You can take heart that it's not your fault, it's the carb's fault. The evil Carbohydrate possesses your body and takes over. It's no longer you deciding what to eat or what is best for your health, it is the carb. It jacks up your blood sugar, giving you energy that you think is going to sustain you to get you through the day. But then, like the evil dog that it is… drops you flat. Leaving you hungry, tired, and scrambling for more. Where is that muffin? That candy bar? Any high carb, sugary food that will make you feel better for the moment until the next meal? And don't kid yourself, that bag of chips is pure carbohydrate disguising itself as a vegetable. Unfortunately those innocent little slices of potato will bring along surges of insulin, the presence of which invites fat to move in and take up residence at your waistline.

Dr. Ron Rosedale, founder of the Rosedale Center, co-founder of the Colorado Center for Metabolic Medicine and founder of the Carolina Center of Metabolic Medicine calls a potato a "big lump of sugar". He goes on to say, "That's all it is. You chew a potato, what are you swallowing? Glucose." He goes on to ask "What is a slice of bread? A slice of sugar." Rest assured that even a piece of whole grain bread, as brown as it may appear, is white on the inside. And it will begin its debauchery, forsaking its healthy disguise, and start to melt into simple sugar right in your mouth. It will continue to transform its healthy appearance into its real sugary self in your digestive tract. Leaving you unfulfilled once again.

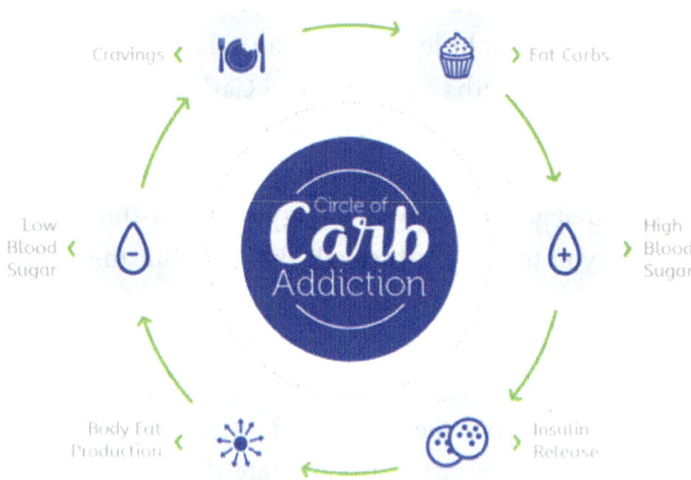
Circle of
Carb
Addiction
Cravings
Eat Carbs
High
Blood
Sugar
Insulin
Release
Body Fat
Production
Low
Blood
Sugar

In the Circle of Carb Addiction, the only thing we have control of is that moment when we "Eat Carbs". If we do that one thing, our blood sugar will go up. If we don't eat them, things will be different. Once we eat carbs, our body takes over and will decide how much insulin to produce, based on the amount of carbs we ate and our individual insulin sensitivity. At the risk of repetition of the chapter on insulin resistance, I will say it all again in a more concise manner. The more sensitive we are to insulin, the less our bodies make. The more resistant we are, the more insulin we need to make. And the more work we cause for our beta cells, the insulin producing cells in the pancreas. If they get overworked, they will wear out before their time, and leave us with an overworked, understaffed pancreas. If we make too much insulin, not only do we have too much sugar in our bloodstream, but too much insulin as well. This is the plight of the Type 2 diabetic. The insulin can't open the gate to the cell to let the energy in, and the sugar in the blood gets too high. Fat is stored.

People experience low blood sugar (hypoglycemia) due to this over-production of insulin. When too much is produced, blood sugar drops too low. It is low blood sugar that triggers that shaky feeling, and drives you to eat carbohydrates. In my experience, people don't realize that hypoglycemia is not just a benign event that means you need to eat. It is a sign that you are overworking your blood sugar management system and need to give it a break.

As a Type 1 diabetic, I manually inject insulin to process even small amounts of carbohydrate. Occasionally, I take too much insulin for the food I have eaten, and it makes me go "low." Hunger ensues. And I'm not talking about just any hunger. It's bone-deep hunger that drives me to the pantry to devour any and all the food in sight. I know firsthand how it feels.

When I feel this intense desire to eat, the thing I should do is eat a little tiny bit of carbohydrate with some protein. Like just one slice of apple with some peanut butter. The sugar in the apple will make my blood sugar rise, and the protein and fat will even things out and keep me from crashing again. When I just eat sugar I feel better, but sugar alone will make it rise and then drop me like a rock again.

So what can be done? How can people be set free from blood sugar up, blood sugar down, weight up, weight down? When you're hungry, you definitely do need to eat. And what you decide to eat can be your gateway to freedom!

Me ~ Certified Sugar Addict

I had a pretty balanced diet growing up. My parents believed in living off the land. We ate 90% wild meat; antelope, deer, with the occasional chicken thrown in. Fried, of course. Catfish caught in the deep holes of the Musselshell River. They grew a huge garden and I had to help. Hence my love of the modern American Supermarket! I love picking green beans out of the bin, standing in line to pay, and taking them home to cook. My parents like the slow-motion version. Plant the seeds, water the rows, hoe the weeds, pick the beans, wash away the dirt, snap the beans by hand, and can them. Canning was a day's work, with the steam bubbling up in the glass knob atop the pressure cooker, jars, lids, and rings lined up and ready to fill, seal, and process. Whew. It was a healthy way to grow up though! The gardening activity I hated the least was picking strawberries. Although it can be hard on a kid's back, you at least get to snack on something sweet while you work. Corn, beets, pumpkins...we grew it all. I hated growing it, and didn't like eating it any better. Learning to like vegetables has been like a really long road trip and I'm still on the journey.

With all this healthy childhood nutrition, it was junk food wonderland when I moved away from home, leaving the country life and embracing the city. My first job was waitressing at the Kit Kat Cafe. More home cooking, but this time with homemade cinnamon rolls, not just occasionally like at Mom's house, but EVERY DAY!!! I discovered the hot fudge cake at JB's Big Boy, my friend Ronda from beauty school worked there and snuck us free ones on a regular basis. Might as well slap that ice cream right on my thighs, as that's where fat lands on my body. Gain a few pounds, buy new jeans.

After that I was hungry all the time. By sheer willpower I was able to keep under the 200 pound mark. I was raised in a different time than now, a time when a smaller percentage of the population was overweight; I think society was less accepting of people who didn't fit the skinny mold. Even though I wasn't technically obese, my weight kept me from the job I wanted.

Almost finished with beauty school, I walked into the most beautiful salon I'd ever seen. I saw eight beautifully dressed stylists in ridiculously high heels… and I desperately wanted to work there. The mirrors were surrounded with Hollywood dressing room light bulbs and the place reeked of modern. My life on a cattle ranch in Eastern Montana was a complete contrast, another world. I liked this one a lot better. I knew my outfit was not up to par, and felt pretty intimidated. When the owner sat down to interview me it was over before I knew it, and I had a feeling I didn't fit in. He was as nice as he could be to a fat girl wearing the totally wrong colors, and encouraged me to get some experience and come see him in a few years. Ironically, I would share an apartment with one of his salon managers a few years later when I was a few pounds thinner. Her name was Dawn, and she took me under her wing, helping me dress for another interview. I'll never forget the outfit I wore. A purple peasant blouse with puffy sleeves, a white skirt with a wide ruffle, a white leather belt with silver Conchos, and white cowboy boots. Hey, it was a look! Dawn thought I looked fantastic and set up a time for me. The owner was much friendlier this time, and offered me a job. I left ecstatic.

My joy diminished in a big fat hurry when Dawn told me I would be making 5 dollars an hour, and that the owner had said, "Help her stay on her diet." WHAT??? Like I needed that amount of stress for that amount of money. Was he kidding??? I met with my accountant, who was my best friend's boyfriend. He himself had transformed his life, losing 100 pounds in a year. He knew how I felt. We went over my current income and analyzed the hit I would take financially. Would working in that environment make me any happy, thinner, or richer? I decided no.

I stayed at the salon where I was working, Family Hair Trends, for six years. I worked with another girl named Kim. She was thin. Loved to run. We didn't have a receptionist, so we took turns leaving our clients to answer the phone. One summer day it was my turn and the person on the other end of the line asked for Kim. I responded with "Which Kim would you like an appointment with?" I expected to hear my name, Kim Ferch, or hers. Instead I heard, "The heavy set one..." Ouch. I think sarcasm took over and here's what I felt like saying, "I'll see if I can find the chunky little pig and get her on the line."

That was it. My "Why". I wouldn't stand for it. I never wanted to be described as "the heavy set one" again.

I began my day without breakfast, who wants to begin adding calories any earlier than you have to? Then when the hunger pangs kicked in I would start drinking diet soda until I finished work, and then hit the drive-thru or grocery store, and eat alone. If nobody saw me eating maybe it didn't count? I don't know exactly how this happened, but for more than 2 years not a single soul saw me eat. When I occasionally would take a bite of pizza somebody ordered for the lunch room at work, some well-meaning, thin, self-appointed food police would say "That's not on your diet!" So I just didn't let them know I ever ate a thing!

There was an all-purpose store across the street, Gibson's Department Store. I bought chocolate covered raisins, orange slices, peanut butter cups...hid them in a cupboard in the back, and snacked to my heart's delight, only when nobody was looking. At night I'd drive though the dark streets of Billings Montana, hit Bob's IGA to find ice cream, doughnuts, hot fudge, M & M's... bursting into tears as I snuck my "food" to my car, wondering why the checker had to comment on my "interesting selection" of items. Fortunately the diet of sugar-free gum and diet soda I enjoyed during the day kept my weight under control. This night-time binging, probably brought on by a day of starvation, ultimately caused my weight to creep up and my self-esteem to creep down. Finally, with a morning weigh-in that shocked me, I decided to do something about it!

You guessed it, a "liquid" diet. By this time I was pretty much afraid of food, and knew that eating made a person fat! I had heard of the Cambridge Diet, and secured my cans of powdered food. Just add water. 21 days, 17 pounds… gone. And I'm proud to say I never gained it back. BUT I am sad to say that I continued my love/hate relationship with food for 25 years.

Not long after I had lost the 17 pounds, I decided I had to kick the gum/soda/doughnut habit once and for all, and joined two of my friends at their home, to take a run at a "cleanse." You may have heard of it. Every morning you mix a gallon of water with lemon juice, pure maple syrup, and cayenne pepper. A very spicy lemonade of sorts! The three of us lived on this concoction for ten days! Eight pounds thinner and very, very hungry, I was a happy camper. I didn't eat another donut or drink a soda for years to come. And I didn't gain the 8 pounds back. I guess I'd have to say I was a successful "dieter", as most people that lose weight gain it back, plus some.

Further attempts to achieve my goal weight took me to a high-fiber diet, sprinkling unprocessed wheat bran on oatmeal and potatoes, and baking high-fiber muffins with ripe bananas and honey, all of this in an attempt to feel full longer and lose the next 20 pounds. I joined a gym, and would ride my bike to try and burn extra calories.

The gym was a huge challenge for me, and didn't last long. In the 80's we were seeing jazzercise, aerobics of all kinds, and spandex. People were getting weighed under water to check their percentage of body fat. One particular day I watched a five-foot nothing blonde prance around the gym bragging about her 17 percent body fat. I remember walking out of the gym, eyes burning with tears as I biked my way home, feeling like it was virtually impossible to achieve the beauty standard that I wanted so badly!

It was during this period in my life, my mid-twenties, when I saw my first Atkins Diet model. My roommate, Eileen, was flipping bacon every morning, making eggs, burgers, steaks, and I watched in disbelief! I said, "Eileen! What the heck are you doing?" I watched her cook bacon with judgement in my heart, as I sat in the dining room snobbily eating my dry baked potato with no butter sprinkled with unprocessed miller's bran. Even as she lost weight I was convinced she was killing herself! I was into "low fat and whole grain." Does that include low fat muffins? We all want to believe that it does.

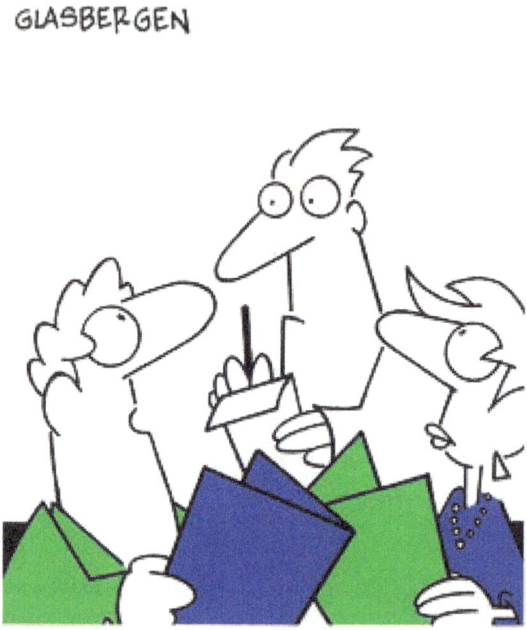

"I'll have some heart disease, high blood pressure and diabetes with a side of clogged arteries and tooth decay."

I managed, through sheer discipline and the ability to live hungry after binging, to maintain a normal weight throughout my 30s and in spite of two pregnancies, be pretty content with my weight. At 40 I had overcome my issues with exercise, and had a personal trainer that showed up every Saturday morning at six o'clock. I had to be there, no matter how late I stayed up on Friday night! I walked 3 miles every morning, and another one or two at night. My girls were 3 and 6 years old, I ate their portions and it was working! I looked good, but I was still hungry most of the time. I bought some "skinny jeans, "an unbelievable size 7. If they fit I was happy with myself and if they didn't, I was bummed. I would begin a starvation diet again until I could get them on!

I would like to say that using a piece of clothing as a gauge is not necessarily a bad idea. I think it is a better way than holding yourself hostage with numbers on a scale. But if your self-esteem is tied to your size, it is not a fun way to live. On the flip side, I'm not sure fat and happy belong in the same sentence. If you struggle to get into your clothes or an airline seat, it isn't a good thing. If you have experienced either of these problems, it doesn't have to be this way. There is hope!

CHAPTER 6

Burning Fat for Fuel

There are two foods the body can use for fuel, carbohydrates and fat. Fat provides energy without causing an insulin response, and it provides a long steady stream of energy that lasts far longer than any amount of carbs will produce.

How to Get to a Fat Burning State...Ketosis

To get ourselves into fat-burning mode, the first thing to do is take away the carbohydrates that give instant fuel. Without sugar available, the body will begin to burn the fat instead. It sounds simple, and it is! One thing to be aware of when switching to low carb, is that our kidneys release sodium and water more efficiently when we eat this way. A high carbohydrate diet, on the other hand, causes us to retain water and salt. Because of this, it is important to replace the salt to avoid feeling weak, fatigued, constipated or headachy. One efficient way is to drink a cup or two of chicken broth each day.

Ketosis is a fancy word for burning fat for fuel. This fat can come from your own personal stores and from eating fat. It is often confused with ketoacidosis, which is not healthy, but can only occurs when blood sugar is over 240 and ketones build up to dangerous levels in the body. Diabetic ketoacidosis develops when Type 1 diabetics don't take enough insulin, causing their blood sugar to soar. Occasionally it can occur in uncontrolled alcoholism, starvation, or from an extremely over-active thyroid. Some folks have heard the word ketoacidosis, confuse the two, and write off a great tool for body composition progress. While the state of ketoacidosis is indeed, dangerous, a healthy low carb diet won't cause a problem.

If you are following a well-formulated high fat low carb eating style, there is nothing to be afraid of. Ketosis is a beautiful thing. It is a natural state, and when you don't eat fast acting fuel in the form of carbohydrates, your body burn fat for fuel instead. In addition to helping you burn body fat, ketosis makes you feel less hungry and helps you maintain muscles.

In order to get off the roller coaster of pounds up/pounds down, I have adapted my body to burn fat for fuel. Following this plan I have no cravings or ravenous hunger, more stable blood sugar, more consistent predictable readings on my monitor, and less fear of complications and life-threatening low blood sugar. Eating this way, people with diabetes can reduce or discontinue blood sugar lowering medications, normalize their weight, and have more energy! People with prediabetes can stall or prevent developing diabetes. People with insulin resistance can halt the production of too much insulin, and change their body composition for the better. Does this sound too good to be true? Trust me, it is possible!

You will find that you can go much longer between meals, with an added benefit of less cooking and cleaning up! It will take a paradigm shift…converting from the notion that we have to eat 5-6 small meals throughout the day to eating less often… but what a relief to not have to carry around snacks everywhere you go! And the glory of not being hungry all the time makes the effort of a little mindset shift totally worth it.

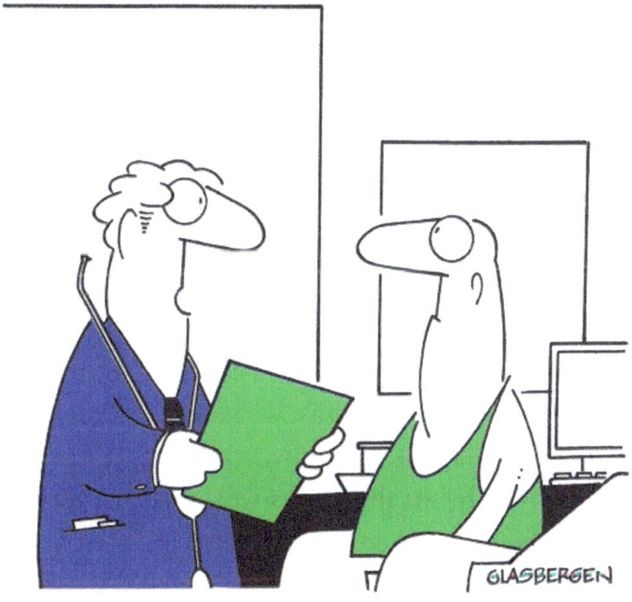

"The good news, it's OK to eat butter after all. The bad news, it's not OK to eat any of the things you like to put butter on."

As diabetics, whenever we talk to a doctor or even a friend and mention any health related challenge, they automatically blame our diabetes for any number of situations. This is a concept known as "anchoring," and can be applied to any stubborn mindset that affects how we process new information. I think it applies to our conditioning around the LCHF way of eating. By definition, anchoring is "a cognitive bias that describes the common human tendency to rely too heavily on the first piece of information offered when making decisions. During decision making, anchoring occurs when individuals use an initial piece of information to make subsequent judgments, not accepting new data."

Dr. Julien Seifter, a nephrologist at Brigham and Women's Hospital in Boston and a Harvard Medical School professor says this about anchoring, "Beyond the ease of retrieval, there's a sense of reward and confidence in going with your first instinct. In addition, there is always a temptation to reach an absolute conclusion, an undeniable thrill in the "aha" moment, as well as a profound satisfaction in unambiguous belief. Then, after we come up with a clever diagnosis that ties together a complex of symptoms, we may be very reluctant to retreat from that diagnosis, even when the negative tests start rolling in."Dr. Seifter wraps up his words on anchoring with these thoughts. "One thing we can control, starting now, is our self-awareness. Become aware of your own biases, let go of fixed ideas, and keep an open mind." More and more new information is rolling in about how detrimental the low fat message has been for people in our world.

> *"I looked at him nonplussed. I realized that I have spent so many years being on a diet that the idea that you might actually need calories to survive has been completely wiped out of my consciousness. Have reached point where I believe nutritional ideal is to eat nothing at all, and that the only reason people eat is because they are so greedy they cannot stop themselves from breaking out and ruining their diets."*
>
> *Helen Fielding, Bridget Jones's Diary*

Science is showing in study after study that low fat is not working for us, that our bodies can and do efficiently burn fat for fuel when allowed to. Because of our conditioning, however, it takes a serious mental adjustment to think it is okay to incorporate more fat in our diets. Doctors are not the only ones susceptible to anchoring, we all are! We hold fast to an idea that we believe in, even in the face of documented new information. The anchor I'm talking about is "we get fat because we eat fat." Our generation was heavily influenced by the "low fat" message. In 1977 when the United States Government issued a mandate that all Americans over the age of 2 should restrict their fat intake, an anchor was thrown overboard that has held us captive ever since. If you listen to people around you, in the grocery store, on the news, on you tube videos, in hair salons (my personal pulse on what's happening in the world), on newscasts… you will hear enlightened well-educated people slip in the words "low fat." It has wormed its way into our subconscious minds due to decades of propaganda based on misinformation; that eating fat is inherently bad and we should eat less of it.

Eating Fat is Fabulous

It is extremely good to know that findings from studies and research are all pointing us to the truth. One of the most significant studies took place in Spain and was reported in April 2013 issue of the *New England Journal of Medicine*. For about five years University of Barcelona scientists followed 7,447 people age 55-80 with risk factors of heart disease, including overweight, smoking, and diabetes. These people were divided into three groups and carefully counseled to follow three distinct diets. 1/3 of the group ate low fat, 1/3 ate a Mediterranean diet which included eating fat, moderate beef, and 1/3 cup of nuts. Lastly, 1/3 of the participants ate a Mediterranean diet as well, but instead of nuts added 4 tablespoons of olive oil. They ended the study early because the low fat group was suffering more heart attacks, stroke and death. It was considered too unethical to continue.

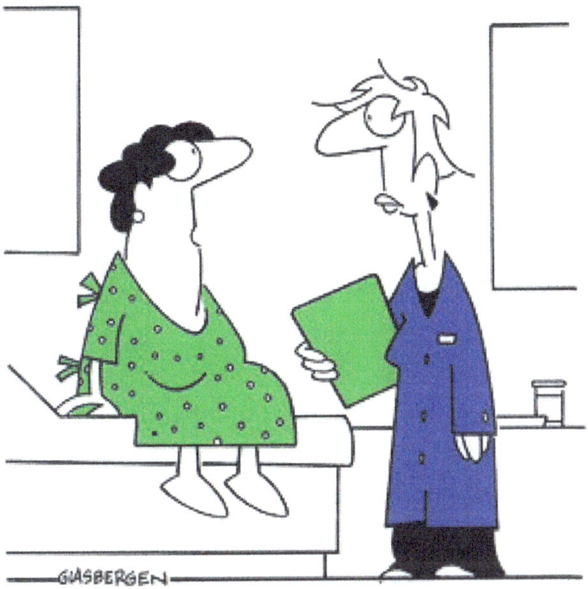

"The Mediterranean Diet is supposed to be very healthy. Can you write me a prescription for a vacation in Greece?"

Dr. Ramon Estruch, a professor of medicine at the University of Barcelona and his colleagues have changed their own diets and are following a Mediterranean one. Dr. Estruch said, "We have all learned."

The Miracle of a new Approach

I know I've said it before, but I am going to say it again. Eating more carbohydrates means the body needs more insulin. Fact of life. Insulin…Fat Storing Hormone. Dr. Stephen

Phinney & Dr. Jeff Volek, authors of *The Art & Science of Low Carbohydrate Living*, tell us, "Insulin turns off fat oxidation and stimulates fat storage." When people are diagnosed with prediabetes or diabetes, the doctor will tell them to lose weight and exercise. Exercise has many benefits, and helps increase sensitivity to insulin which means the beta cells don't need to make as much to keep up. But the lion's share of the problem is better managed by what we eat. It is impossible to exercise enough to counteract a carbohydrate splurge. Your blood sugar goes up when you eat carbs, and the surplus of insulin produced shoves the excess glucose into the cells to be stored as fat. If you get nothing else out of this book, I want you to understand why we store fat. Understanding leads to a better chance for life-giving change.

> *"I did then what I knew how to do. Now that I know better, I do better."*
> *Maya Angelo*

I am grateful for doctors, scientists, and researchers who are leading the way for us to understand and use food to feed our bodies and make us healthy. Dr. Stephen Phinney is a physician-scientist who has spent 35 years studying diet, exercise, fatty acids, and inflammation. Dr. Jeff Volek is a professor in the Department of Kinesiology at the University of Connecticut where he leads a research team exploring the physiologic impact of diet, exercise, and nutritional supplements. These experts give us hope for better health through education. Here are two of their documented observations:

1. There is a "dramatic reduction in serum triglycerides seen in individuals with metabolic syndrome who go on a low carbohydrate diet."
2. We have "multiple observations that a host of biomarkers of inflammation go down when a low carb diet is adopted."

I am often asked the question, how many carbs are too many? How many carbs should a person eat in a day? Volek and Phinney tell us that some people with metabolic syndrome might be able to lose their symptoms at 100-125 grams of carbohydrate per day. But someone with diabetes, who has been consuming around 300, might need to cut his carbs to 20-25 per day. If people will do it, the doctors say in their experience "this has caused the diabetic, in only a few weeks,

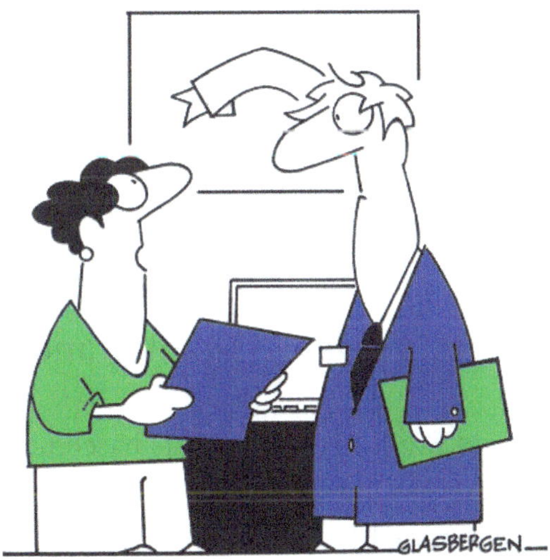

"Too bad it was a typo. I was doing pretty well on the low-crab diet."

to free themselves of insulin injections, oral medications, and at the same time experience better blood sugar management."

Mark Sisson, author of the *Primal Blueprint*, has a similar message.

300 or more grams/day – Danger Zone!

Mark says in his blog, "www.marksdailyapple.com" that this amount of carbohydrate will deliver a high risk of excess fat storage, inflammation, metabolic syndrome, and diabetes.

150-300 grams/day – Steady, Insidious Weight Gain

Continued higher insulin-stimulating effect prevents efficient fat burning and contributes to widespread chronic disease conditions. This range is irresponsibly recommended by the USDA and other diet authorities - this leads to the statistical US average gain of 1.5 pounds of fat per year for forty years.

100-150 grams/day – Maintenance Range

This range *could* work for some people based on body weight and activity level. When combined with exercise, it allows for genetically optimal fat burning and muscle development. Enjoy abundant low-starch vegetables and moderate fruit, and avoid grains and sugars.

50-100 grams/day – Effortless Weight Loss

Minimizes insulin production and ramps up fat metabolism. By eating moderate protein, non-starchy vegetables and mostly berries for fruit (easy to stay in 50-100 gram range, even with generous servings), and staying satisfied with delicious high fat foods (meat, fish, eggs, nuts, seeds), you can lose one to two pounds of body fat per week and then keep it off forever by eating in the maintenance range. I think Mark may be using a broad brush to paint this picture, as it is my experience that most women need to eat closer to 50 or even less for weight loss.

0-50 grams/day – Ketosis and Accelerated Fat Burning

Excellent for intermittent fasting towards aggressive weight loss efforts, provided adequate protein, fat and supplements are consumed otherwise. May be ideal for many diabetics.

Part of the process of burning fat includes making ketones, which are organic compounds that show up in your blood and urine. It is unfortunate that even the medical community is not well versed in this natural process. Not too long ago I went to a walk-in-clinic for a urinary tract infection, because my doctor was unavailable. The nurse practitioner noticed the ketones in the urine sample and showed concern. She was a little surprised by my happiness, and I told her I like ketones and want to have them all the time! I gave her a quick overview of my LCHF eating, and fueled my desire to help someone understand the process. She seemed to be enlightened, anyway.

If you think of carbs as dry grass and fat as a lump of coal, it's a good example of how our bodies use fuel. When you strike a match to the grass, the fire rages across the field, consuming everything in sight. When the grass is gone, it doesn't have anything left to burn, and dies out. This same action happens when we eat sugar filled foods, because they give us a quick-acting source of energy. When we've used it up, we are completely out of fuel, and crave even more. If, instead, you set fire to a bed of coals, the fire produces a steady burn, with fuel to last for hours on end. You can find in-depth information on fueling our bodies and in particular for exceptional athletic performance in the book *The Art and Science of Low Carbohydrate Performance* by Drs. Steven Phinney and Jeff Volek.

Phinney and Volek are top docs when it comes to the science behind the LCHF strategy and have documented evidence in the book. Many athletes are embracing their philosophy, and are utilizing long acting fuel to achieve superior performance; no more "hitting the wall" and needing to constantly carb-load to keep going.

Researchers are conducting more and more studies and the evidence is definitely mounting for using fat as our fuel of choice. We are seeing the benefits not just for diabetics, but for anyone who wants to manage their weight, have more energy, and perform at a high level of endurance.

The Nirvana of Fat Burning

How do you know if you've reached Ketosis? The Nirvana of Fat Burning? We've talked about the fact that when you are burning fat, your body produces ketones. The most common way to confirm they are there, and you are on the way to changing your body for the better, is to test the urine. When you are just getting started in the ketogenic lifestyle, it is a good feeling to see the tip of a ketone stick change color and know you are producing ketones. It helps keep you motivated and committed. It isn't the most accurate, but it is worth using in the beginning. After our bodies become keto-adapted, the body efficiently burns fat and therefore sluffs off less ketones; the urine won't show as much action. For this reason, if people are depending on the stick to change color, they feel like they are losing their fat burning state, when in fact they are not. There are just less ketones present in the urine.

Ketone urine testing strips are small plastic strips that have a little absorptive pad on the end. The pad contains a special chemical that changes color if there are ketones in the urine. The container will have a scale on the label, with blocks of color for you to compare with the strip after about 15 seconds. Follow manufacturer's directions.

Ketone test strips can be purchased at any pharmacy for around $15.00, and are usually kept with the diabetic supplies. In some stores they're kept behind the counter, but don't require a prescription to purchase. If you don't see them on the shelf, just ask the pharmacist.

To really get a good picture of your body's level of ketones, you can buy a blood ketone tester called Precision Xtra (from Abbott) which Jimmy Moore, Author of *Keto-Clarity* says is the most accurate and consistent.

There is a breath ketone analyzer, new on the market, called Ketonix. It has shown to be as accurate as blood meters, doesn't require strips and you don't have to poke your finger! A Swedish engineer, Michel Lundell developed the device and was a finalist in the 2014 Shark Tank Competition for epilepsy management innovation. Michel's interest in measuring ketones comes from the fact, that he is an epileptic. There has proven to be a great reduction in seizures when people with epilepsy follow a LCHF diet. In fact up to 50% less. Before anti-seizure medicine was invented, high fat diets were commonly recommended. While this isn't the subject of this book, it is interesting to note that there are other physical challenges that can be addressed by eating this way, including heart disease. Dr. Helen Hilts told me she has seen fatty liver resolved in as short as two weeks on low carb! Studies are currently being done on its effect on Alzheimer's and Parkinson's disease.

CHAPTER 7

The Magic of Muscle

by Fitness Trainer Andrea Hall

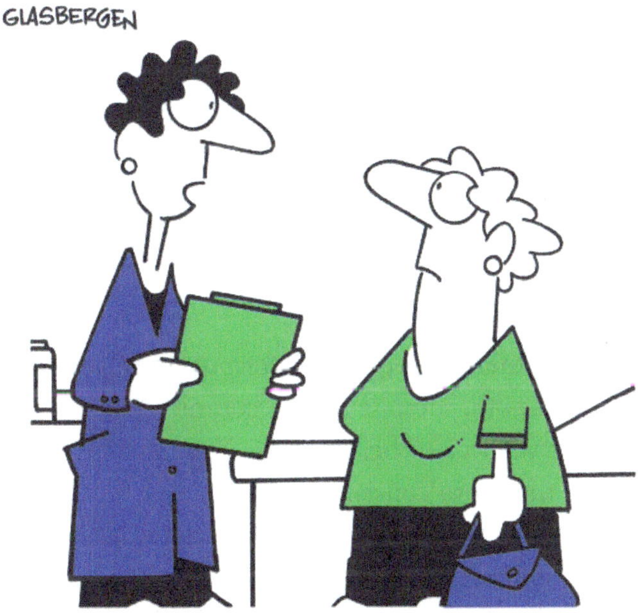

"What fits your busy schedule better, exercising 30 minutes a day or being dead 24 hours a day?"

"The keys to overriding the decay code are daily exercise, emotional commitment, reasonable nutrition, and a real engagement with living. But it starts with exercise." Wise words by Dr. Henry Lodge in his best-selling book, *Younger Next Year*. Every day that we are not working on improving our health, our bodies slowly decay. As we age, our bones, joints, and muscles lose density, strength and size. Our mobility and balance suffers and our nervous systems crash.

But don't freak out just yet! Exercise has compound effects that can reverse the "decay code" and create an even better, more fulfilling life. Strength training and HIIT, which we will cover soon, have many anti-aging mechanisms that can fight disease, improve the strength and condition of your body, fight disease, increase insulin sensitivity, restore damaged metabolism, and of course, burn fat! People who exercise regularly also have greater stamina as they age, manage pain, have improved posture, and decreased risks of injury.

Unfortunately, there is no quick-fix formula to achieve physical fitness and health, despite what commercials and social media might want us to believe. The benefits of exercise are cumulative, the more consistent you are and the longer you participate, the better you will feel. The best way to transition into this healthier lifestyle should not really be a transition at all. It should be an immediate, sharp break from the old and an instantaneous decision to embrace the new. Once you have made that decision you will see things begin to change, and I'm not just talking about the size of your pants.

It should be an immediate, sharp break from the old and an instantaneous decision to embrace the new.

The next time you hit the gym, take a minute to let the euphoric feeling after a good work-out sink in. This sensation is not just a short-term effect. It is proven that your body continues fighting off tension, anxiety, anger, and depression after exercise! As a result, you will begin to notice that along with your regular exercise routine will come an overall improvement in your general well-being; because once you feel good, you do good, and you also look good! Exercising gives you the strength, optimism, and flexibility to take on life like you never have experienced before!

Research shows that people who are physically active and maintain a healthy weight, on average, live about seven years longer than those who are inactive, overweight or obese. It is *your* body and you are the one that has to live in it! So if you treat it nice, you have a much better chance of it treating you nice right back. Exercise is one of those habits, when we incorporate it into our lives, can positively affect almost every other area and lead to success!

So, you might be thinking, "What kind of exercise should I be doing? How often should I be doing it?" My training strategy consists of two parts: high intensity interval training, also known as HIIT, and strength training.

HIIT consists of alternating periods of short bursts of high intensity exercise coupled with rest periods of low intensity exercise. This is done back and forth for a set number of rounds, distance, or time, depending on the program prescribed. The main determining factors for engagement in the program are:

1. your current physical condition
2. your goals
3. what kind of activities you enjoy

HIIT can be applied to running, biking, swimming, hiking, and many more. The importance lies in the alternating levels of intensity.

An example is as follows:

1. Warm-up: 10-15 minutes working up from low to medium intensity for 5 minutes either running, on the elliptical, stepping machine etc.
2. Work Interval: Increase intensity to at least 80% of your maximum heart rate using a combination incline, resistance, and/or speed. Hold at this rate for one minute.
3. Rest Interval: Drop down to a low to medium intensity of 40-50% of your maximum heart rate and hold for two minutes.

Rounds: Repeat 5-8 times

Cool-down: 5-10 minutes using an easy level of exertion

HIIT is the most beneficial form of endurance exercise because in addition to increasing the state of the body's cardiovascular health, it is a fat-blasting mechanism! It increases the excess post-exercise oxygen consumption, meaning that generally for about two hours after the workout, the body is still burning energy to restore itself, increasing the overall expenditure by about 15%! To reach the maximum benefits of HIIT, you should do it at least two or three times a week.

However, HIIT is only part of the equation. Strength training is equally, if not more important. Strength training involves the use of resistance to induce muscle contraction in order to increase strength, the size of skeletal muscles, and the body's anaerobic endurance. With my clients, we go over how to properly perform each exercise and gradually increase the intensity to guarantee the significant benefits that building muscle has on the body. There are three reasons to build muscle that I am going to focus on... and you will see what I mean, they're magical!

More Muscle Means Less Fat

When you combine your new eating habits with an effective strength training program, your results will be even better!

Most people still think that aerobic exercise is the best way to lose fat, but recent studies show that it's muscle that really contains the magic! People spend hours and hours doing cardio every day when they could be spending three hours a week on strength training and getting even better results. Having more muscle means that you burn more calories all day every day for the rest of your life.

Each pound of muscle that you gain burns 30 to 50 calories each day in addition to what is already being burned! This is because muscle is an active tissue; it needs fuel to function. Your muscles are magical because they are able to tap into fat stores and use them for energy! Think about it. If you replace five pounds of fat with five pounds of muscle, you will increase your metabolism by 10%, causing you to shed unwanted fat and create the body shape that you've always desired to have. So, what do you think sounds easier? Burning a few calories while you're running on the treadmill, or burning more calories continuously by gaining muscle?

Muscle Sensitizes Insulin Receptors

Not only is strength training great for swimsuit season, but it also improves blood-sugar and insulin sensitivity, which further explains why gaining muscle burns fat. As we discussed earlier, insulin is a hormone that drives blood-sugar or glucose out of the bloodstream and opens the gates of our cells to be used for energy. Whenever carbs or protein are consumed, insulin is secreted by the pancreas and released into the bloodstream. When excess amounts of glucose are ingested over extended periods of time, the body becomes insulin resistant and can no longer open up those gates to each cell to be absorbed and used. Instead, sugar floats freely in the bloodstream, raising blood sugar levels until it is stored as fat.

Here is where the magic of muscle comes into the picture. Muscle fibers are lined with insulin receptors, and once the insulin attaches to those receptors the gates are opened. This allows excess glucose to enter muscle fibers and be used for building muscle! As you tear down your muscle fibers through weight training, they must rebuild to grow bigger and stronger. As you stimulate your muscles and force them to rebuild, they absorb and use excess energy that has been stored during the process. Because resistance training signals the glucose floating around in your blood to enter the muscle cells, it increases insulin sensitivity. Strong, toned muscles burn glucose more effectively, which helps regulate blood sugar even when you aren't moving.

Strength Training Modifies your Mood

As we discussed earlier in the chapter, exercising is more than just a physical experience. It's a psychological experience. To explore how resistance training modifies your mood even further, we'll look at how the body functions on a biological level. When you exercise, your body releases endorphins, which are chemicals that interact with the receptors in your brain to reduce pain perception. Endorphins affect the body in a similar way that morphine does; they trigger positive feelings in the body.

Regular exercise truly does have therapeutic effects. It has been clinically proven to reduce stress, fight off anxiety and feelings of depression, boost your self-esteem, and even improve sleeping patterns. According to a study published in *Psychosomatic Medicine* in 2000, researchers separated 156 significantly depressed adult volunteers into 3 groups. One group was given antidepressant medicine, one did 45 minutes of exercise three times a week, and the final group did both medicine and exercise. After four months, all three groups saw equal improvements in their moods. But the amazing thing that was discovered, is that after another 6 months, 38% of the medicine takers fell back into depression, 31% of the medicine/exercise group relapsed, and of the group that exercised only, the relapse rate was a mere 8%. When you feel good you perform better, and as you perform better you will have a much more positive and energizing outlook on life!

These mood improvements can partially be attributed to increased blood circulation to the brain from exercise, which has an influence on the HPA (hypothalamic-pituitary-adrenal) axis, and therefore on the physiological reaction to stress. The HPA axis also communicates with the limbic system, amygdala, and the hippocampus. The limbic system controls mood and motivation, the amygdala responds to stress with fear, and the hippocampus plays an important role in the formation of memories as well as motivation and mood. You can see how the brain has the ability to significantly affect how we feel!

The brain has the ability to significantly affect how we feel!

Strength training and HIIT are vital to your health, especially if you have struggled with unwanted weight or have been diagnosed as diabetic or pre-diabetic. It is a natural way to improve blood glucose, increase muscle, tendon, ligament and bone strength, and improve overall quality of life.

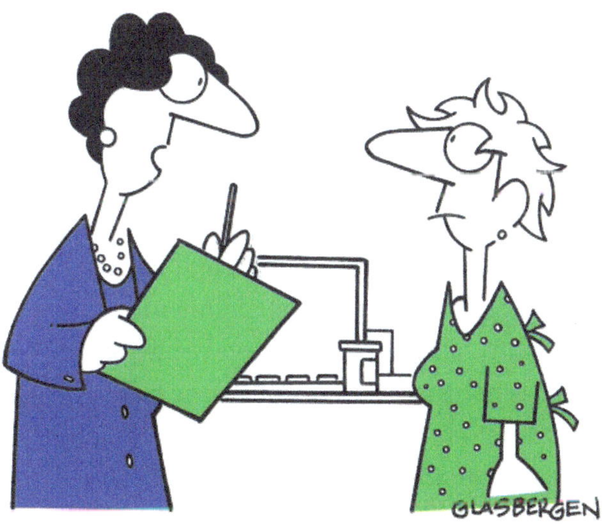

"Resistance training is just as important as cardio. Train yourself to resist chocolate, pastries, fried foods, beer, pizza...."

Getting Started

It's easier said than done, I know. The weight room can be intimidating when you first walk in. You will see strong, physically fit people and feel they will judge you. The equipment may look complicated and confusing to use; but there are ways to turn this fear into excitement. Here are three steps that can set you free from fear and doubt as you embark on your journey to physical fitness:

1. **Find a trainer.** Get some one-on-one help with a qualified fitness trainer that can address your goals, assess your limitations, and teach you how to correctly move and position your body safely to avoid injury...AND doing exercise correctly will help you get the best results you can.

2. **Go with a friend!** Having someone to motivate and encourage you can actually be the difference between success and failure. It can also give you the confidence you need to get in the gym and try out new things, and even give you a little competition to push your imagined limitations and perform to your best ability. The accountability is a plus as well. When my mom started her most successful run at fitness, our neighbor came knocking on the door every morning at 6:00 am. The knock came...she went to the gym!

3. **Think long-term.** Try to get away from thinking in the short term. Commit to a long-term process and the results

will come. Living a healthy life doesn't have to be hard. Your new normal can be going to the gym every week. It's not a sacrifice or an obligation, it's just normal. When you commit to being consistent over the long-term, you might be surprised and actually see remarkable results in the short-term. Set a schedule for your training and "just do it!"

4. **Make it a priority.** Don't do it just when you feel like going or when it's convenient. I will tell you right now, it's not going to get done and you will not see the results you want. Put your workouts on your calendar and organize your life and responsibilities around them. There will always be emergencies, of course, that will prevent you from your gym time; that's life. But if you schedule your training when life gets busy, you won't miss one work-out that ends up turning into missing 4 weeks of workouts.

5. **Reward yourself.** What you are doing deserves regular and repeated rewards! Give yourself some credit! Buy yourself some new running shoes or allow a little extra time to relax throughout the day. It's not just about the number on the scale, it's about consistency and motivation to keep going and triumphing over your own personal physical and mental blocks.

In general, I prescribe 3 days of weight training per week and two days of HIIT in order to see consistent progress over the duration of each program. The one rule that you need to follow is that you *must* take at least one full day off to recover. At the very most you should be exercising six times a week with a combination of strength training and HIIT.. But again, the frequency and intensity of each work out depends on you, the individual. Carefully assess your condition when you begin, and your goals; which is why you should consult with a trainer to get off to a great start and see results in a timely manner.

I know that there is a learning curve to this new way of life. I was not always in the greatest shape. In fact, I was diagnosed with severe progressive adolescent scoliosis at a young age and had to have spinal fusion surgery to correct it. This put my body through a lot of trauma and it took a long time for me to fully recover. I know how it feels to be weak, unhappy with your body, and intimidated by the gym; but once you make the decision to do it, you just have to do it! Follow the simple steps I've outlined here (be sure to check with your doctor before beginning any new exercise program) and you will be much more confident and happier in the long run. Don't let your setbacks stop you from where you want to go, how you want to feel, and how you want to look. You are on your way to becoming the person you always wanted to be! Start today!

CHAPTER 8

Change

David Byrd, renowned achievement coach tells this story. "Two men were on a sugar-free diet. A well-meaning friend walked up and offered them each a Snickers Bar. One replied, 'I can't have sugar.' The other said, 'I don't eat sugar.'" The point is well taken; a person who sees himself as a victim of circumstances says "I can't." A person who believes that he can affect his outcome in life, that his behavior matters, says "I don't." He takes personal responsibility for his decision to abstain from sugar. If we can change our words we can change our attitude, and changing our attitude gives us improved self-esteem and a feeling of strength and power. The more often we speak and feel from a place of power, the stronger we will become and the better our choices will be.

"I could never..."

I think one of the biggest challenges to changing our eating is our mindset, the way we feel about changing our diets. It is important to create optimism around the opportunity, and embrace the change as a positive experience. Most of us probably think of ourselves as relatively optimistic, but obesity, pre-diabetes, and diabetes are real struggles for many. It can be a challenge to be optimistic when faced with hunger pangs, high and low blood sugar, the constant temptation of "goodies" around every corner, and the fact that we have to make choices that affect our health day in and day out.

Shawn Achor, author of the *Happiness Advantage*. In truth, reality is different for each individual, because reality is altered by perception. The definition of real is how you see things in your perspective. What is real to you. Keep in mind that "real" is a moving target, depending on who's viewing it. It is Shawn's belief, as a researcher and happiness expert, that it is best to accept our circumstances and realize that what has happened to us isn't necessarily what we wanted, nor would we want a similar thing to happen to anyone else. But it did, and it has, and it isn't going away. Every once in a while my husband will say, "I'm tired of being diabetic, I think I'll stop now". He's joking of course, and most of the time keeps an optimistic perspective about being diabetic.

Deciding to Make a Change

The first and most difficult part of changing behavior is coming to the point of decision. What will it take to trigger a change? Will you have to hit bottom? Where is bottom? Consider the man who, with some prodding from his wife, takes enough interest in his health to visit the doctor on a yearly basis. He goes, but every year it's pretty much the same story. Doctor says, "You need to lose some weight, exercise, manage stress". Every year he tells himself he will do better. Deep down he knows he won't, and the doctor knows it too.

But this year is different. Just a few short months after his physical, he felt pressure in his chest. Shortness of breath caused him to alert his wife. As the symptoms continued she rushed him to ER. Thanks to modern medicine and the amazing life-saving cardiac department his life was saved. This time the man surprised his doctor. The double bypass was his "bottom". It cost him several months of missed work, creating a domino effect of extra work for his team as they tried to cover for him. It cost thousands of dollars in medical care, thank God for insurance. Part of the cost included stress on his family, as they worried that he might die. Then there's the depression he faced as he tried to rally and get his former pace back on track. When my own father was hospitalized for over two months with a quadruple bypass, I learned that a high percentage of heart patients experience significant depression following a heart-related incident. This affects the person for years to come, delaying their return to a productive and energy-filled life!

What could have happened to avoid the pain and suffering of heart surgery? Could the doctor have said a key phrase in a certain tone to move the man down the road toward a healthy lifestyle? Could his wife's nagging somehow gotten through to him? Do you think that he really didn't think his daily choices would make much of a difference in the outcome of his health? Or do you think he knew, but found a way to justify just one more French Fry? My hope is that you will see, that daily seemingly insignificant choices can make a big difference. Change is not only possible, it can be easier than you think.

There are two types of people in the world when it comes to motivation, those who are motivated by positive outcomes, and those who are motivated by negative ones. Thankfully, not everyone has to reach bottom! I've also heard the two perspectives called "towards" motivation and "away from" motivation.

The "towards" people, the goal oriented individuals, see a possible positive outcome, and move towards that objective. These are the people that benefit from the "dream board." By making a poster of their desires and goals, a visual picture of their exciting expected outcome, they keep their goals top of mind and continue moving towards obtaining those goals. When temptation strikes, the thought of the end result will intercept their thoughts and cause them to make a decision in the heat of the moment that will help them reach the goal. Swimsuit season is coming and a chocolate chip cookie will delay the desired goal of looking great in a bikini.

The "away from" crowd is motivated by the possible negative outcome, and they will draw energy from thinking about how bad it's going to be if they are pudgy at the beach.

I have two daughters, and they are polar opposites when it comes to their motivational styles. One girl pins up pictures of girls with six-pack abs and swimsuits, and is proud to say after 2 years of hard work she has her own rippling abs. My other daughter has lost 30 pounds, and gains her motivation from the dire consequences of being overweight. She looks at overweight people and old photos of herself for motivation, and says, "Mom, I'm not going back there!"

It doesn't matter what gets you moving and keeps you going, as long as it works for you. If you aren't sure which to choose, choose both! Make the dream board. Put a screen saver on your computer of your desired positive outcome. Think about what will happen if...and push yourself over the decision-making cliff with whatever it takes. My friend Laura, who coaches people for a living, says that in her case (and I would assume in your case as well), making the decision is the challenging part. After you've firmly decided what to do, picked your motivating mindset, and decided HOW to proceed, doing it is a whole lot easier.

In his book *The Happiness Advantage*, Shawn Achor gives a great tip when it comes to making decisions. He calls it "the 20 second rule." Here's how it works. Make your new behavior easier to get to than a less desirable one. If it takes you 20 seconds longer to make a wrong move, you may be more apt to make the right one! He gives this example: Put the batteries to the remote control for the television in a drawer, where it will take more energy to get them out and channel surf than it will to read a good book! Put the book on the end of the sofa, where it's easier to get to than the remote. Put healthy snacks within reach, veggies chopped and ready to eat, and hide (throw away and don't buy more) the potato chips. Make sure you have to expend considerable energy to get to them. Our natural instinct is to take the easy way, the smooth road, so work with your natural instincts! Make sure the things you know are good for you are much easier to do than things you will regret in the morning! I was fortunate last year to hear Shawn speak, and he said in his talk that once you have your gym gear on, your mind perceives it is easier to just go to the gym than to change your clothes; for that reason he sleeps in his gym clothes!

Changing things starting with behavior seems logical, in spite of the fact that it is commonly perceived that true and lasting change must come from the inside. Outside change could be seen as phony, trying to look like something that you're not. I agree that it is not in our best interest to live a lie or try and cover up who we are to impress the world. I believe in authenticity. However, fake it till you make it has some merit. For true change to happen on the inside, the behavior on the outside can lead the way.

Fake it till you make it!

If you want to know what changes you need to make to lead you to your goal, find someone who has already achieved a similar goal and adopt the behavior of that person. Why re-invent the wheel? When I met Dr. Hilts and heard her story of change and how she had overcome Type 2 diabetes with low carb, I thought, "If she can do it, I can do it!" I have to change my behavior to change my life.

It is far better to make a sharp break
with the past and a serious
commitment to the future.
Chris Crowley

As Americans we are surrounded by food choices, take a good look around any grocery store and see what I mean. The aisles are filled with so many choices it is completely overwhelming. Just the breakfast cereal aisle alone is insane! Those foods are on the outside of us, each one vying with every marketing strategy possible, to get us to put them into our mouths, swallow, and make them part of us. Inside your body is your precious blood, carrying oxygen to your cells, energy to your muscles, and keeping you alive. We need to make a shift on the outside in order to live a healthy life on the inside.

Eating LCHF (Low Carb High Fat) is becoming a part of who I am. I am a diabetic who is achieving normal blood sugars in order to live healthier and longer and not suffer and die from complications. Sure, some things have to change, but trust me, it's worth it! I'm worth it. You're worth it!

Making a Commitment to Change

The Ah Ha Moment, the Reality Check, the Light Switch goes on. You finally have arrived at the place where "I've had enough." It's when you know that you know that you know that you want a better life. A healthy life. But how do you get through the maze of information. Who is Right? There are the Vegans, the Vegetarians, the Paleos, the Atkins People, the Protein Power People, the Medi-fast people, the Zone Diet People, the Weight Watcher's People, the Raw Food People, the Mediterranean Diet people. And you know as well as I do, that there are thousands more. Everybody touting a plan to help you lose weight and get healthy. So why should you believe me? Why don't you try it and see? Dr. Andreas Eenfeldt, a Swedish physician, says in his You Tube video, *The Food Revolution*, that you can try this way of eating on yourself and don't have to even read all the science, unless you're into that sort of thing. If you want detailed scientific information from and expert, go to "www.dietdoctor.com/science."

If your doctor has mentioned you need to lose weight, "keep an eye" on your blood sugar or get some exercise, you could be pre-diabetic. If you're not there already you could be on your way. If you struggle with weight or have been a yo-yo dieter there is a viable solution. Even if it's just a few extra pounds you wish you didn't have, this is a glorious way to live. I personally have lost 11 pounds, and the good news is they are the last 11! The clothes in the closet are all the same size, and the doctor says my weight is good. What a change, after 35 years of gaining and losing.

Looking back on my diabetes, I wonder what if I had remained unaware of my situation. Remember, my three-month average blood sugars were well within what the medical establishment likes to see. But when I looked at the chart of a "well controlled" (like me) diabetic who used a continuous glucose monitor, there were clearly extreme highs and lows. It was time to change. I followed my doctor's advice and made over the pantry and the refrigerator. I made a master grocery list and stocked up on great high fat, low carb, moderate protein meals and snacks.

Dr. Eenfeldt posted a video on his website spotlighting a physician in England, who left his practice to actually move in with his patient. Dr. Rangan Chatterjee spent two months with an out-of-control diabetic man and his family. The doctor felt the husband was a walking time-bomb for a heart attack, and really wanted to help the man. After agreeing to the program, the family went on a low-carb diet with intermittent fasting and some high-intensity interval training. The result of his program…the family called it a revelation! In just two months his blood sugar control was massively improved, he went off most of his diabetes drugs and lost all the weight he needed to lose.

What if, as a person who should make changes, you don't do it? Of course, that is the case of many of us, and statistics show what happens when we don't. As a diabetic the consequences are dire. There are plenty of good reasons to control blood sugar: eyesight and kidney function to name two.

I am so glad I made the decision to adopt LCHF eating, because It feels good to look at my average blood sugar and know I am doing everything I can to take care of myself; for me and my family. The side benefit of staying a consistent normal weight is now motivating me as well. For several years I have had more confidence in my appearance and my ability to manage not only my diet but my life. (With the exception of the piles of mail in the office). I couldn't have guessed this weight and size stability would be such an added benefit at the onset.

Whatever your motivation, running away from obesity and the associated health risks, away from a genetic pre-disposition to diabetes, or away from low self-esteem and constant regret, it's time to make the decision to change! And if you're running towards better health, consistent numbers on the scale, an outer image that corresponds with your new inner confidence, all the better.

If you are struggling with the idea of changing what you eat, ask yourself the following questions:

1. Is my health where I want it to be?
2. Where will I be in one year if I don't change a thing?
3. Where will I be in one year if I follow a diet low in carbohydrates, high in healthy fat, and moderate in protein?
4. What obstacles stand in my way?
5. How can I deal with each one?
6. What substitutions can I enjoy instead of carbohydrate choices?
7. Why should I do this?

If you are not sure you can do it, spend some time considering that it might be possible. Motivational speaker Les Brown has a talk on the power of possibilities. He teaches that if you cannot make a positive statement like, "I eat low carb high fat," take a baby step and whisper, "It's possible." I believe that any attempt to eat fewer carbohydrates will result in health benefits for you. I also believe it is harder to try and cut back than to make a clean break from fast acting carbs like sugar and grains. As far as "cheat days" go, keep them to a minimum. Would you tell a former smoker that he can have a cigarette every Sunday? Absolutely not. We all know that just one could trigger a return to the habit of smoking. The longer we abstain from our trigger foods, the less we crave them. Fewer cravings, fewer opportunities to compromise and slip over the edge... back into the cycle of carb-addiction madness.

If you are ready, I believe you can most certainly do this! Many people have gone before you and their stories are strikingly similar. Get involved in the online low carb community and you will hear countless stories of weight loss, dependable consistent energy, normal blood sugar, and other benefits you would never expect.

I'm asking you to make your highest, realistic level of commitment. I say realistic, because it is better to set a reachable goal and achieve it, than to set an unrealistic one and fail. Achievement Coach David Byrd says in his Achievement Success Program, "goals are meant to be achieved." Not like your typical New Year's Resolution that is made year after year, with very little planning and an underlying feeling that you will never actually do it.

It is very important to do what you say you are going to do, even if you don't tell another soul about it. Because when you break your word to yourself, you lose credibility with guess who, yourself! Everything you decide to do is then met with skepticism. "Really?" you say to yourself. "Just like you lost weight last year? Just like you went to the gym last year?" And the self-doubt persists until you are so beaten down that you flat out can't tell yourself you are going to make any changes at all.

My cousin Nick Winter wrote a book called *Motivation Hacks.* (Read it, you'll like it) I smile when I read it, because I know first-hand how far he has come. I knew him before he changed his life. His change was based on creating "success spirals" for himself. After reading about motivation and success spirals in the book, *The Procrastination Equation* by Steel Piers, PhD. Nick devised his plan and created goals around many things he wanted to achieve, but felt he wouldn't because he was so consumed with work. These goals were designed to be so small that he absolutely knew he wouldn't fail. After putting together a string of small victories, he was able to move on to bigger and more substantial goals that allowed him growth in many areas, physically, mentally, relationally, and in his businesses.

After you make a commitment, put together a plan for success. Look at your kitchen, your habits when dining out, your work schedule, your family. Sit down and have a conversation with yourself or a friend or a counselor about your feelings surrounding food. What are your long standing beliefs and do they need to be re-evaluated? Are you convinced that you have to eat a low fat diet to lose weight? Do you think you need to experience hunger to be thinner?

I assure you that your decision to restrict fattening carbohydrates is the right decision. I am told that the reason doctors and dieticians don't tell their patients to eat low carb is that they don't believe people can do it. I don't agree. The friends who have contributed their stories to this book don't agree. They've done it, I've done it, and You Can Do It Too!

We don't have to live a roller coaster life of pounds up/pounds down. I don't have roller coaster blood sugar, I experience more consistent predictable readings on my monitor, and have less fear of complications or life-threatening low blood sugar.

It really is possible.

CHAPTER 9

Emotional Eating

Where are you now?

Where do you want to be?

How can you get there?

A typical question in my house is, "What do you feel like having for dinner?" With the typical response, "I don't know, what do you feel like having?"

Because eating and what we decide to eat is closely tied to our feelings, it is a worthwhile activity to journal your food for a week and add your feelings to the journal. This will tell you whether you are eating to satisfy physical hunger to fuel your body or emotional hunger to numb your pain. If you haven't had much experience in recognizing feelings, this will be an excellent exercise in getting to know yourself. Don't be afraid to honestly acknowledge how you feel. In order to help you, here is a list of feelings for you to choose from. How much easier can it get?

If daily journaling every bite of food seems overwhelming,

make a list of the foods you typically eat in a day and then on the weekends. Close your eyes and think back, attach a mood to a particular food or time of day that you eat.

Moods

Enraged	Disgusted	Surprised	At Ease
Livid	Pessimistic	Energized	Calm
Anxious	Despondent	Pleased	Relaxed
Repulsed	Miserable	Pleasant	Mellow
Panicked	Depressed	Upbeat	Sleepy
Furious	Hopeless	Cheerful	Easygoing
Frightened	Disappointed	Lively	Secure
Apprehensive	Discouraged	Happy	Chill
Troubled	Lonely	Joyful	Thoughtful
Stressed	Sad	Festive	Complacent
Frustrated	Disheartened	Motivated	Content
Angry	Exhausted	Enthusiastic	Satisfied
Worried	Apathetic	Focused	Restful
Concerned	Bored	Hopeful	Peaceful
Tense	Tired	Exhilarated	Tranquil
Nervous	Ashamed	Inspired	Loving
Irritated	Bewildered	Optimistic	Grateful
Uneasy	Cautious	Proud	Blessed
Shocked	Cynical	Playful	Comfy
Restless	Embarrassed	Elated	Cozy
Annoyed	Guilty	Excited	Fulfilled
Aggravated	Hungry	Thrilled	Touched
Grumpy	Numb	Blissful	Balanced
Hysterical	Overwhelmed	Confident	Carefree
Jealous	Rejected	Determined	Serene
Rushed	Restless	Flirty	Blissful
Smug	Suspicious	Refreshed	Accepted

Date	Time	Food	Mood

It's one thing to decide what you feel like having for a meal, and another to be overwhelmed with a feeling, seek out comfort food and dive headlong into a binge. Or pull up a movie and sit in despair munching away an entire bag of chips or popcorn.

The good news is that once you've made the physical adjustment to LCHF (Low Carb High Fat), your physical cravings will not be a factor. Another piece of good news is that there is a new ketone supplement on the market that helps convert your body to fat burning state in record time. (www.mynewbff.pruvitnow.com) It is astonishing what can happen when our bodies are running smoothly and efficiently on fat, have plenty of energy, and aren't crying out for nourishment on a cellular level. No more cravings that cause intrusive thoughts of food…or one big thought of food that lasts from morning to night.

At the extreme end of the weight loss scale, I recently heard of a woman who lost 270 pounds, and she declares that she did not crave food and was not hungry when she ate LCHF. She met Dr. Eric Westman and he told her that her weight was not her fault…knowing that fact helped her cope with emotional baggage, let go of guilt of overeating, and begin to heal. In fact, Dr. Westman's program for people who suffer is called HEAL, which stands for Healthier Eating And Living. His program is designed specifically for Type 2 Diabetics who want to live healthy lives without prescription medicines and needles, and it also can prevent diabetes and promotes weight loss without hunger.

There is a lot of support out there as we move forward towards a new saner existence when it comes to food. It helps me to know I am not alone. There are people who have been where I have and are a few steps ahead on the journey.

www.dietdoctor.com

www.livinlavidalowcarb.com

www.healclinics.com

www.marksdailyapple.com

www.garytaubes.com

Breaking the Hold of Addiction

I believe that many of our emotional eating issues are additionally complicated by addiction issues. I know I was addicted to sugar, and felt like what I ate was out of my control. Most of us do have food cravings. According to the journal, *Appetite*, 97% of women and 68% of men report experiencing them.

We hope that satisfaction and happy feelings will be the result of consuming an enjoyable food. I'm not sure "satisfaction" is how I would describe my ability to eat four apple fritters in one sitting, sick to my stomach was probably more like it.

It's just that for me at that time, one fritter wasn't enough.

We are all one of a kind. You are different from your mother, your best friend, even your twin sister. You are created to be you, special and unique, and unlike any other. Some of us can have a glass of wine or two, unfettered by the addiction that causes another to have a drink and begin a downward spiral to the bottom. Even though the addict may have experienced the joy of sober living for a period of time, something tips them over and they clutch a bottle again, letting go of their progress and heading down the road of destruction one more time. In kind, some can eat toast for breakfast without heading for the donut shop and succumbing to a binge that lasts long enough to tip the scale to some number that triggers despair. Then they are overwhelmed with the feeling; "I've done it again... WHY???"

It important that we know our personal limit when it comes to eating carbs. It is referred to as our Carbohydrate Tolerance. It differentiates the skinny-minnies who seem to float through life eating bon-bons and whatever else they seem to want and stay thin and at least look healthy on the outside from those with extreme carbohydrate intolerance, who gain weight by walking into a donut shop. My friend Marilyn told me that she doesn't go near pure sugar, ever. She said "I respect sugar like I respect deep water." Good analogy.

The guy who needs to be very cautious is the no holds barred "carbaholic." That was me, and if that is you too… I am so sorry! We are the ones who, like the alcoholic who shouldn't take that first drink, shouldn't eat the first donut hole. It's because our craving takes over like an alien possessing the brain, or in some cases as dramatic as a demon, causing us to do what we said we'd never do again. But we did it anyway. Because we HAVE to, we CAN'T stop, and FLAT OUT just can't help it.

That's why, even though to some it may seem silly, we need a program of recovery. There is clear scientific evidence of sugar addiction and cravings. When giving talks on food, I always get a laugh when I refer to my twelve-step program. It is funny, since food is a legal substance, and hardly considered something to need recovery from. But folks who are caught up in the cycle of addiction to sugar probably aren't laughing. The pain is real, and if you are feeling that pain and hurt, eating for other reasons than legitimate hunger, you can attend Overeaters Anonymous meetings for support. My brother and I went to one to see what it would be like, and the care and concern was obvious. Each person defines their own "drug of choice" and what abstinence means to them. They learn to avoid trigger foods and reach out to a sponsor when tempted. How awesome to have social support while getting healthy instead of social pressure to continue eating "food" that is ultimately going to make you sick.

As in other recovery programs, such as Alcoholics or Narcotics Anonymous, slogans are used for affirmation and to help keep folks on the right track.

The Use of Slogans

Using slogans has helped me tremendously. I learned some from friends and made up some of my own. Any words you put together, memorize, and that follow the guidelines below can become a slogan.

Hughes & Stuart, a leading marketing firm, published their top criteria for slogans. Their 10 rules may help you create or choose slogans that work for you.

A Slogan

1. Is a simple, direct, concise, crisp statement
2. Defines a new reality or way of life
3. Inspires action
4. Delivers the promise of transformation
5. Makes you think, but not too hard
6. Adopts a distinct personality of its own
7. Is both timely and timeless
8. Is universal
9. Sounds good
10. Is easy to remember

We have all experienced being caught up in a negative or angry repetitive thought pattern. This way of thinking can be particularly unpleasant and often damaging. Like a cow chewing her cud, we bring up past events, attach meaning to them which may or may not be true, and ruminate for hours. Our thoughts spin around in our brains, sucking the life out of the moment and stifling the future. By interrupting and replacing those thoughts with a positive, life-affirming slogan you will not only break the negative cycle but create and reinforce a new flow that is both beneficial and positive.

It is not necessary to investigate the old thoughts, simply notice them, acknowledge their existence, and replace them. If you do want to explore your past, it is a good idea to work with a counselor or really good friend who can help you find truth and meaning in the events of the past and move on quickly. My work with women over the past 35 years has taught me the futility of wallowing. It seems to just cement the negativity even deeper and prevent positive personal growth. On the flip side, I have witnessed good results when clients write about the past or hurtful events in their lives and attach meaning to them. What lesson needed to be learned? The writing process allows us to begin to get clarity and closure.

Christine Caine, founder of A21 ministry which rescues girls caught up in sex-trafficking, is a world changing visionary and thought leader. She gave a sermon recently at my church. She asked us, at the end of each day, to think about our train of thought during that day… how did it affect our day. How do we feel as a result of what we thought about? Did we maintain our joy or were we filled with worry? Do we wonder, "How did I get here again?" and then realize it's because we got on the same old train again. She challenged us to "lay new tracks" in our mind, it's the only way we can arrive at a different mental and emotional destination. She added in closing that the rapidly advancing science of neuro-plasticity, (which means that we can continue to grow and expand our brains and mental capacity), is confirming what God has said all along. We have the ability to change the way we think. Romans 12 says, "Be transformed by the renewing of your mind." It would be great if we could just download new thought processes or push a magic button. Instead it is a management issue, with an ongoing need to catch the wayward persistent way of thinking and coax the train onto a new track.

Slogans are an effective tool that helps to make that shift. Brain studies show that neural pathways are either strengthened by repetition, or weakened by lack of use. By replacing negative thoughts with a slogan, you can literally rewire your brain while at the same time weakening habitual negative and unproductive thinking.

Deborah McNelis, owner of Brain Insights and award winning author of the *Brain Development Series* states, "Repetition is exactly what the developing brain needs. When experiences are repeated, the brain creates strong pathways of connections, and the brain *retains those connections*."

When you feel the motion of a downward emotional spiral, a slogan can not only break the habitual pattern, but also replace it with a positive emotion. Slogans are the ultimate mobile device, you can use them anytime, anywhere. Whether in the car, at work, with friends, or on your own, you can benefit when you think your slogan in your mind. Saying it out loud is even better, as you not only think it, but say it and hear it. Saying and hearing make it a physical experience, making the words even more powerful.

Using a positive slogan repeatedly is a form of meditation. The Bible gives us excellent guidelines for thoughts we should consistently think and meditate on.

> *"Whatever is true, whatever is honorable, whatever is just, whatever is pure, whatever is lovely, whatever is commendable, if there is any excellence, if there is anything worthy of praise, think about these things"*
>
> *Philippians 4:8*

When you realize that your thoughts have wandered into negativity, as quickly as you can, grab a slogan that meets the criteria, and refocus.

Twelve step programs highly recommend the use of slogans for effective change in addictive behavior, and have since their inception in 1935. Studies have shown that almost twice as many alcoholics are abstinent after 16 years who went to AA meetings than those who didn't go at all. I'm sure there are many other factors that contribute to the success, including the support of people on the same path and spiritual growth, but the friends I have who experience successful recovery are active users of slogans. Let's use them!

Choose from these or make up your own

Carbs make you hungry, fat keeps you full

Eat fat to burn fat

It's not my fault, it's the CARB's fault

I eat when I'm hungry, stop when I'm full

Drink when I'm thirsty!

Think...think...think

One day at a time

Let go and let God

This too shall pass

Expect miracles

If it works, don't fix it

Health is a journey, not a destination

Live in the present

We are only as sick as our secrets

Be part of the solution, not the problem

Keep an open mind

Willingness is the key
Let it begin with me
Just for today
Before I say, "I can't" say, "I'll try"
God is never late
I am not alone
Getting healthy for me
Look for similarities rather than differences
Count my blessings
Share my pain
Let go of old ideas
Replace guilt with gratitude
Change is a process, not an event
I take what I want and leave the rest
Help is only a phone call away
I can't give away what I don't have
Anger is one letter away from danger
I have courage to change
Easy does it
Bring the body and the mind will follow
The first step in overcoming mistakes is to admit them
Formula for failure: Try to please everyone
When I do all the talking, I only learn what I already know

Don't make decisions when Hungry, Angry, Lonely, Tired (H. A. L. T.)

I'm not required to LIKE it, I'm only required to DO it

Time wasted in getting even can never be used for getting ahead

I am exactly where God wants me to be

My control is limited to my own attitudes and behavior

Just for today I will live through this day only, and not tackle all my problems at once

There are two days in every week which I have no control over, yesterday and tomorrow

"Be here now, be someplace else later.
Is that so complicated?"
David Bader

I wish I could push that magic button and heal the hurts that drive us to devour food in an attempt to alleviate pain. It is such a strange thing, to look back and see how I used to constantly think about food, crave food, and devour food. Strange indeed, but true. I actually thought I was getting back at someone else by gorging myself! I'll show them! Like the saying, "Crazy is drinking poison and expecting someone else to die."

I remember a situation with a hairdresser I worked with in 1983. She was tall, thin, and worked in the last styling station in the row. This station was directly in front of the swinging doors that led to the break room. Those doors were usually open, and if she caught me eating she took it upon herself to tell me that whatever I was eating was not on my diet. I would say nothing, but her words would trigger a binge, and when she wasn't looking I would dive into my secret stash. Candy Corn, Chocolate Covered Raisins, Nestlé's Crunch Bars…as much as I wanted of whatever I wanted. So There. I showed her!

This is craziness at its finest. What possible injury am I inflicting on her by eating myself sick? What emotional wound am I treating in myself by acting this way? If you find yourself trying to feel better by eating copious amounts of food, I completely understand. Weren't we all raised with our moms giving us treats to make us feel better? Or to motivate us. Or to celebrate. Let's face it, food has been our companion in almost every activity or situation in life. And some of us keep hoping it will make everything better, no matter how many times it lets us down.

Instead of turning to the pantry, there are alternatives. The recent research and developments surrounding brain science have given us wonderful insights into healing emotional wounds. You can find some inspirational and educational short talks on the subject by going to "www.ted.com." TED stands for Technology, Education, and Design, and you will hear talks from leading thought leaders who challenge us to consider new and different ideas. I found 9 talks on Ted dealing with the subject of emotional pain, and ways of dealing with it. One of my favorites is "Why we all need to practice emotional first aid" by Guy Winch. His book is very good...*Emotional First Aid: Healing Rejection, Guilt, Failure, and Other Everyday Hurts.*

In his Ted Talk he compares our tendency to immediately treat a physical wound with proper medical care to our lack of treatment of emotional wounds. He gives particular attention to loneliness, which was one of my biggest reasons for eating. For over ten years I lived with roommates, most of whom seemed to have more going on than I did. Even though I was active in my church, successful at work, and had a lot of friends, it seemed like they were all going out on dates, getting engaged, getting married, having babies, and I felt like the fat girl left at home by myself.

*"Our feelings are like a moody friend,
who can be totally supportive one minute,
and really unpleasant the next."
Guy Winch*

Guy describes the thought processes that I endured and many of us succumb to, that lead from emotional pain to even more emotional pain. We get an idea in our head, like NOBODY LIKES ME BECAUSE I'M FAT, and we become convinced the idea is true. According to Guy, "You have to gain control." It is very hard to change our minds. BUT IT CAN BE DONE! "You have to gain control over the situation (how it feels) and break the negative cycle before it begins". (Stop emotional bleeding)

"Our feelings are like a really moody friend, who can be totally supportive one minute and really unpleasant the next."

He goes on to say that a good response to emotional pain is to treat yourself with the same compassion you would expect from a truly good friend. Catch your unhealthy psychological habits and change them. Rumination, he says, is one of the most damaging patterns we have. This discovery takes us back to the slogan. When you are hurt emotionally, you can't stop replaying the painful scene in your head, and if your response to that pain is spending precious time focusing on negative events, you are putting yourself at risk for clinical depression, alcohol or drug addiction, eating disorders, and even cardiovascular disease.

According to Winch, current brain research shows that even a two minute distraction can be enough to break the cycle of perpetuating a negative thought process,

Battle Negative Thinking

- Take Action when you're Lonely
- Change your Response to Failure
- Protect your Self-Esteem
- Heal your Psychological Wounds
- Build Emotional Resilience

This is not just a battle in your mind, it is a spiritual battle as well. In my early 20s I found myself in a counseling session with the pastor of my church, who also struggled with his weight. It definitely helped me to know that even someone I looked up to as a strong spiritual leader had a similar problem. I wasn't alone, and it didn't mean I was a bad person. (If only we had known about low carb!)

What he did know, was that I was caught in a bad place, and starving and binging wasn't healthy for me. The popular wisdom at the time was all about a "high fiber" diet, and I embraced it. I went to a health food store and bought unprocessed miller's bran. I ate it every day, on baked potatoes, on salad, in muffins. For the first time in a long time I was eating real food, and feeling full for a while. The binging began to dissipate as I started to eat regular meals with people watching.

It was a perfect situation for me to live with my parents again, knowing that they loved me and didn't judge me for eating. For almost two years I had been a "closet" eater, not a single person on the planet had seen me eat. I couldn't bear the thought of people commenting about my eating habits. I distinctly remember my good friend Marilyn saying to me, "Kim, I have never seen you eat." And I thought, "Yep, and it's going to stay that way!"

Pastor Benson gave me a Bible verse to consider and I made a slogan out of it, Colossians 2:16. "Let no man judge you for what you eat or drink." I meditated on it and let the message become part of my psyche. I began slowly by eating in front of my parents, and gradually other close friends. I eventually got to the point where I could eat at work, knowing I was becoming stronger. I realized that what other people thought of my food and bodyweight was not going to tip me over and send me on a trip through 3 drive-thru windows and a stop at the grocery store.

When you decide to make changes in your life around the food you eat, people will question what you're up to. When you stop eating sugar, especially foods that turn to sugar like potatoes and bread, it could raise a few uneducated eyebrows. It is fairly popular to be "gluten free" right now, but LCHF is still relatively new in the game.

Keep in mind, though, that it's your own health that matters most, and if people are really your friends they will understand. We in the low carb community hope that freedom to choose a Low Carb High Fat lifestyle will spread; word of mouth, friends telling friends, family members supporting each other in healthy choices. We can turn the obesity boat around, help diabetics manage their blood sugar, reverse complications, and above all, set people free from the emotional food bondage in which many have been living.

Chapter 10

I Got My Life Back... Vicki's Story

During the last 10 years of my life, I have spoken to many people about diabetes and the challenges they face. No one's story has touched me in the way this one does. It is real, true, and gut-wrenching. A dramatic story of life with diabetes, and the peace that comes when a person comes to terms with their disease.

Understanding leads to a better chance for life-giving change. Seeing those changes sparks hope!

Vicki was born and raised in my home state of Montana. A happy little girl with 2 younger sisters, Patty and Connie. The trouble began when her mother died of cancer at the young age of 41, when Vicki was just 14 years old. Her father, overcome with grief at the loss of his wife, became so depressed he couldn't work and ultimately took his own life at the age of 42. Devastated, the three girls went to live with their dad's sister. Looking back at her dad's life, Vicki can see that both diabetes and depression ran in his family. She didn't escape the genetic combo.

"I was hypo-glycemic my whole life. In high school I would get shaky, eat a banana, and feel okay again. Later, I remember having my hair shampooed in my salon and feeling so weak and shaky I couldn't get out of the chair. The stylist had to run next door and get me bananas.

"I vaguely remember a doctor mentioning to me that I was pre-diabetic around age 38 in the mid 1980's. But he sure didn't make a big deal about it. Funny, but the only guideline I remember him giving me was to eat bran muffins. Pretty bad advice as I know now!

"At age 41 I was diagnosed with depression. Physically though, I felt fine. I was thin. Then just four years later, during a routine physical, that same doctor casually said, 'Well…with your diabetes…'

"SHOCK! He had never officially given me any reason to be concerned about developing diabetes! Seeing the surprised look on my face his only comment was, 'Well, you've been pre-diabetic for a very long time.' My parents had died so young, I couldn't have known about the genetic predisposition. It certainly was there, because both my younger sisters developed diabetes. In fact, my sister Patty and her husband are both diabetic.

"The doctor said, 'You've got to get this under control,' but I didn't go to any education classes. I bought a meter, and went through periods when I'd be a perfect little diabetic. Then I would get distracted by life and stop paying attention. My weight was up and down.

"The roller coaster blood sugar lifestyle that I lived definitely took a toll on me. Looking back I can see that the way I managed my diabetes was in direct correlation with life events and the stress that ensued.

"My Aunt and Uncle have a daughter, and she is like a sister to me. Laura became a dietician at University of Montana, and after her time working in a hospital decided to become a Diabetic Educator. She currently owns and operates her own business called Take Control in Missoula, Montana. She and her team provide health coaching services for weight loss, pre-diabetes, diabetes type 1 and 2, and gestational diabetes along with helping people with other positive life changes for healthy living. Multiple times in this journey I have called Laura for sound advice. She was always there for me when I called for help. I remember when my sister Patty was diagnosed. Laura tried to work with both of us over the phone. It was the early 2000's and I got off all my medication because I was eating so well and exercising. But then a crisis would come up and I would fall off the wagon. It was always a case of not paying attention and eating to feel comforted. I didn't partake in drastic binges like my sister Connie did. She would buy a cake and eat the whole thing! It must have been hard on Laura to watch the cousins she loved like sisters go through so many ups and downs, knowing what diabetes does to the body. She had flat told me on many occasions what I needed to do.

"My down times were not a reflection of knowledge of the disease. They were a direct result of either denial or being in such a stressful situation I could not think of myself at all. One of those times was when my sister Connie was diagnosed with colon cancer.

"Connie was very private and didn't want to be the center of attention, so her best friend and I were the only ones that knew. The burden of keeping it all inside weighed heavily on my heart. Keeping up the façade, I would lie when people asked me about her appearance, because I vowed to respect her wishes. . I took her to chemo and did the best I could. Her diabetes was discovered a few months before she died, and was secondary to the situation we were in.

"I spent every moment I could with my sister as her health declined. Six weeks before she died, my husband left me and moved out of the house. I knew things weren't great, with me spending all my days off taking care of Connie. He worked too many hours too. I tried to reclaim my time-starved marriage, but he declared that it was too late.

"Now what was I to do? Living in Seattle, I had become weary of the clouds and rain. After spending a year in counseling and working up the stamina to make a move, I decided to move to a sunny climate.

"Arizona has proven to be the place where my health has become a solid focus and the birth of a new life. It took some time to adjust, though. I was excited to move to a warmer climate, but didn't feel good when I arrived. The first 6 months I felt so tired and drained, I slept most of them and was unable to even look for a job. At 65, with the ups and downs of life and diabetes, it took some time to get off the sofa! My weight was totally out of control, I was eating candy and all kinds of other things I shouldn't have been eating. For some reason it didn't even occur to me that how I felt was partly my diabetes!"

The Big Change

"The big change all began with a doctor's appointment. I knew I had to find a local doctor, and had seen this one a couple of times. I told her I was in control of the diabetes, (I don't know what I was thinking!) but how could I have been? The trigger for me to even see a doctor was that I was SO thirsty! She ordered a fasting blood sugar test. BLOOD SUGAR CRISIS! That's what she said to me. She said I was going on insulin that very day. (That was my Ah Ha moment.) My A1c was 13.5. I was experiencing blood sugar averages of over 400.

"Devastated by having to take insulin, I asked her if I would be on it for the rest of my life. She said, "That depends on if you do what I tell you to do." This response finally got the message through to me, that if I wanted to live and be healthy, without a heart attack, stroke, blindness, or kidney disease, it was really and truly up to me and my decisions. In May of 2015, at the age of 65, I took responsibility for my life and my health for the very first time."

"I did then what I knew how to do.
Now that I know better, I do better."
Maya Angelo

"I've lost 40 pounds since May. I started with 30 units of Lantus, a long acting insulin, with a goal of dropping the units gradually to 10. I'm there! As my diet became low carb, my blood sugars began to normalize. My morning blood sugars are 90-115. My A1c is 7. My cholesterol is normal and so are my triglycerides. My doctor is thrilled, and I feel good. Throughout the day I am able to maintain steady and near normal blood sugar. The one missing piece is exercise, and I think I'm ready."

The day I got that report I felt like I could fly.

"I was ecstatic. I called the people that matter to me the most.

I felt like I had accomplished something in my life just for me. Knowing I did it gives me the enthusiasm to move forward. At age 65, I have a new lease on life…it is not an understatement to say, I got my life back."

CHAPTER 11

Eight Obstacles to Low Carb

I know how you feel. I've been there, and have to do it every day, just like you. It would be so much easier if we could say, "Say No to Eating" and go about our day. And like my daughter said when she was five… "That settles THAT problem!" Unfortunately it's not that easy. We are confronted every day with food images in our own minds, and we are pummeled daily with images and messages from advertisers.

Just for fun, take a look at the most remembered Super Bowl Ads from 2012.

1. Doritos (Grandma slings baby across yard to grab chips)
2. M&M's (M&M shows his milk chocolate)
3. Doritos (Dog buries cat and bribes owner with chips)
4. Sketchers (Gorun: Little dog moonwalks across the finish line)
5. Coca-Cola (Polar bear has trouble catching bottle of soda)
6. Bud Light (Dog fetches drink at the mention of his

name)
7. Pepsi (Sir Elton John is dumped into the king's dungeon)
8. Budweiser (End of Prohibition to now…beer-fest)
9. Go Daddy (Danica Patrick and Jillian Michaels body paint a model)
10. Budweiser (America celebrates the end of Prohibition)

In order… we have chips, candy, sneakers, soda, beer, soda, beer, beer, domain hosting, and beer. People! What is our world coming to???

But does watching and remembering these commercials actually make people eat more junk food? Research from Cornell University and published in the journal *Appetite* found that food and beverage ads really do increase cravings for those specific products. As it turns out, watching cooking shows does too!

This is the world we live in on the outside. And then there's the world within. All the memories about food, the comfort gained from eating certain food items, the holidays, the birthday parties, the traditions. With all this working against us, there are 8 obstacles to LCHF that will try to prevent us from having success. Knowing these obstacles allows us to prepare adequate strategies, both offensive and defensive.

OBSTACLE 1
You're afraid to eat fat.

It seems to make logical sense that eating fat will make you fat. And as you have read, this theory has been overwhelmingly supported by health professionals and our government. According to Gary Taubes in his book, *Why We Get Fat*, the belief that dietary fat is the cause of heart disease led directly to the idea that eating carbohydrates would *prevent* it. Science has proven that this is not true. Oatmeal is not a heart-healthy food! Eating fat is a healthy way to live, and hopefully this book has helped you feel better about it… and even better about burning it. If we cannot overcome our fear of fat, it is impossible to sustain this way of eating. Our bodies need fuel, and without carbohydrates or fat, we can't make it through the day. Decide today to choose fat!

What kind of fat should you eat? Experts recommend that your primary fat choices are olive oil, coconut oil, butter and full-fat cheese, avocado and nuts, and you can eat seafood, fish, pork, beef, lamb or chicken (even the skin).

OBSTACLE 2
You believe there isn't enough variety in low carb food choices.

I don't know if I can convince you that this is a lie, because a trip through any grocery store has way more food choices than we need, as a matter of fact it is darn right overwhelming. The average grocery store has over 300,000 items. The thing to do is run towards the positive, good things that you love and are good for you, and run away from the carbs! Take a look at the foods listed in Chapter 12 and highlight your favorites. If you like to cook, the possibilities and combinations are extensive. When you see someone chowing down on something that isn't on your list...ask them, "Can I have a bite of yours?" You will find that just a bite will satisfy your taste buds, give you some variety and won't destroy your weight loss efforts or your blood sugar control.

Obstacle 3

You believe you can't give up your favorite foods that have carbs.

When I was in college we were required to read a book for a psychology class called, *Telling Yourself the Truth*. This book was a complete life-changer for me. It challenged me to look at my beliefs, and "mis-beliefs". The following story from the book has stuck with me for over 30 years. Perhaps because I was one of those who believed I couldn't give up donuts and ice cream and cinnamon rolls. I was driven by addiction. I was powerless over food.

Connie, who is 65 pounds overweight, says she can't lose weight, she's helplessly fat. Her weakness is ice cream. We asked her to imagine she was sitting in an ice cream parlour with an enormous ice cream concoction sitting in front of her. Picking up her spoon she is about to dive into the thing when suddenly from behind her she hears someone speak.

"Drop that spoon!" he says menacingly.

She's stunned for a moment. "I said drop it, lady!" The voice repeats. She then feels something cold and hard against her temple. The voice is fierce. "This is a gun, lady, and if you take one bit of that ugly mess, I'll blow your head off."

Connie's reaction is immediate. "I wouldn't eat the ice cream!" she gasps.

"You mean, you wouldn't touch it?"

"I wouldn't touch it!"

So much for helplessness.

Replace the word "Can't" with the words "It's Possible". Because given the right mindset and effective self-talk, ANYTHING is possible!

OBSTACLE 4

You don't believe you can attend a party or holiday event without eating carbs.

One of the biggest temptations in life is a holiday or party, with a vast array of tempting, fattening, carb-infested, foods beautifully displayed right in front of your eyes, staring you down through the entire event. I used to think I had every right to "treat" myself to some of each, coming back for more of my favorites. Even wrapping a few irresistible items in a napkin and sticking them in my purse for later! But having made the decision ahead of time to eat only low carb it is possible to relax, grab a cup of nuts or a plate of veggies and a glass of red wine. Trust me, parties are much more fun. Focus on the people, the conversation, and the entertainment...and you won't go home feeling sick from eating and additionally feeling the need to starve yourself the next day to try and make up for it!

If the event is not formal it is acceptable to contribute something fabulous that IS on your eating plan to ensure that you will have something to eat that you enjoy.

Be sure to eat a snack or meal before you leave home so you don't show up to a party starving. This is a key strategy for me and I rarely ignore it.

When I have parties at my house or host parties for others I have found that people who attend are openly relieved and grateful that there are so many healthy low carb choices.

OBSTACLE 5

You believe it will be too hard to eat different foods than your family/kids.

A high fat, moderate protein, low carbohydrate eating plan is good for everyone in the family. Nobody in my family complains about our tasty marinated chicken or grilled cheeseburgers. Everyone enjoys scrambled eggs and bacon, berries, and nuts. The food list in this book comprises 80% of the food in our house. The other 20%? A few things I buy occasionally to treat the non-diabetics that live here.

OBSTACLE 6
You believe you'll have to give up fast food and restaurants.

Happily, In and Out Burger coined the phrase, "Protein Style" and started a trend of burgers wrapped in lettuce! A delicious option, and available most places I go. If they don't know the verbiage, just describe it for them and they'll do it for you. I also learned from my mother-in-law that you can go to Subway, choose all the meats, cheeses, and vegetables you would normally put in a sandwich, and they'll put it in a bowl and chop it up to make an impressive salad, just the way you like it! I'm sorry I can't give you a terrific replacement for French fries, so the rule applies, "Can I have one of yours?"

OBSTACLE 7
You believe you don't have time to cook/eat low carb.

Zooming around the perimeter of the grocery store should save you time in shopping. You may have heard of that strategy before to help you shop healthy, and it works very well. Most of the aisles are filled with processed packaged foods that are lower in nutrition than fresh whole food. I begin shopping in the produce section, head around to dairy, fresh meat, fish, and seafood, and shopping is almost finished. A few canned or frozen items rounds it out, tuna, cans of chicken and chicken broth, frozen vegetables and berries, almond milk, butter and heavy cream. Quick and Easy!

Kids and Grandmas are good for washing and chopping if you have them; containers of ready to eat healthy snacks and recipe ingredients make meal planning simple and easy. Even if you have to do it yourself it is totally worth it. Consider all the time you will save not going to the doctor for obesity related illness!

OBSTACLE 8
You believe it is genetic, it can't be helped.

Researchers have not yet discovered a specific gene that causes obesity, although several genes are considered to be important in playing a part. Although our genetic make-up can result in a predisposition, the environment plays a much larger role in the likelihood of our becoming obese. You may be genetically susceptible, but you'll be a lot better off without a high carbohydrate diet coupled with a lot of time on the couch. Your genetic make-up, which you have inherited from your parents, contributes to your general body type, including where your body deposits fat. BUT! You can defy your DNA and make a difference in your health by choosing to eat low carb and maintaining a generally active lifestyle.

It is a lot easier to make this change cold turkey than to try and wean yourself. Eating less carbs is like asking an alcoholic to "cut back." He/she/you might be able to maintain for a while, but 9 times out of 10 we give in to the cravings, because the cravings won't go away until the sugar is gone. Can you imagine telling a recovered smoker that it's okay to follow the 80/20 rule? Smoke only 20% of the time and that's good enough? Or just smoke on Sunday?

Before making the ketogenic low-carb decision, are there any reasons you might NOT want to do it? Stare down obstacles and stop them dead in their tracks. When you are tempted, you can look back at the moment you decided to make the change and stand firm based on your past decision.

Design a contract for yourself to sign; you can find a sample in the back of this book. When my oldest daughter wanted to take piano lessons, the teacher wisely suggested that she sign a 6 month contract. This was a great idea because when it came to daily practice and she didn't "feel" like practicing, I just had to remind her that she had already decided to practice every day, and signed a contract. This gave her the impetus to sit down and do what she had promised herself, her mother, and her teacher that she would do.

Find a friend to be your accountability partner. Ask your doctor to act as your witness, or hire a coach...just make sure that you are serious, have considered the obstacles, and planned ahead what to do about them. Choose someone who will stand strong with you, and not "feel sorry for you" and buy you chocolate chip cookies!

Keep in mind when considering these obstacles, that perception is key. How you look at something will completely determine your feelings about it.

CHAPTER 12

What Should I Eat?

What has been is what will be
and what has been done is what will be done,
and there is nothing new under the sun.
Is there a thing of which it is said
"See, this is new?"
It has been already
in the ages before us.
Ecclesiastes 1:9 and 10

The food I eat has been recommended by many people, and for a very long time. In fact, as far back as 1901, William Osler in his book, *The Principles and Practice of Medicine*, advises obese women to "avoid taking too much food, and particularly to reduce the starches and sugars." In 1951, a textbook was published by seven British physicians, *The Practice of Endocrinology* and recommended the following:

Foods to Avoid:

1. Bread and everything else made with flour...
2. Cereals, including breakfast cereals and milk puddings
3. Potatoes and all other white root vegetables
4. Foods containing much sugar
5. All sweets...

You can eat as much as you like of the following foods:

1. Meat, fish, birds
2. All green vegetables
3. Eggs, dried or fresh
4. Cheese
5. Fruit, if unsweetened except bananas and grapes.

When you look at the basic food plan laid out here, the only thing that's new is that I haven't typed it up before. But I'm sure you've read it before in lots of other books, articles, and magazines.

Don't be surprised. There is nothing new under the sun.
Only endless repackagings .
John Piper

Dr. Eric Westman is a faculty member of the Duke Clinical Research Training Team. His research is focussed on disease prevention. Because the two major causes of disease and death in modern society are obesity and smoking, his research involves clinical trials on both.

The following basics are adapted from *The No Starch No Sugar Diet* by Dr. Westman.

Meat: beef, pork, ham, bacon, lamb, veal, sausage, pepperoni, hot dogs, or other meats

Poultry: chicken, turkey, duck, or other fowl

Fish & Shellfish: tuna, cod, tilapia, salmon, catfish, bass, trout, shrimp scallops, crab, and lobster or other fish

Eggs

Salad Greens: 2 cups must be eaten every day. If it's a leaf, it's fair game. arugula, bok choy, cabbage (all varieties) chard, chives, endive, greens (beet, collard, mustard, and turnip), kale, lettuce (all varieties) parsley, spinach, radicchio, radishes, scallions, and watercress

Non Starchy Vegetables: **1 cup a day.** artichokes, asparagus, broccoli, brussels sprouts, cauliflower, celery, cucumber, eggplant, green beans, jicama, leeks, mushrooms, okra, onions, peppers, pumpkin, shallots, snow peas, sprouts, sugar-snap peas, summer squash, tomatoes, rhubarb, wax beans, yellow squash, zucchini

Beef and/or Chicken broth are strongly recommended, because you can get extra sodium along with magnesium and potassium from them. You can get it at most grocery stores, but it's not nearly as good as the broth you can make yourself. You can make it ahead and freeze it! Unless your doctor tells you that you need to restrict your salt intake, do not use low-sodium. Many people have reported that the broth helps them get through carb cravings.

Cheese: Up to 4 oz a day, swiss, cheddar, brie, camembert, bleu, mozzarella, gruyere, cream cheese, and goat cheeses. Check the carbohydrate count.

Fats & Oils: This is the GOOD news! You can even eat butter. olive oil, peanut oil coconut oil... avoid hydrogenated oils and margarine. Chopped eggs, bacon, and grated cheese are great in salads. Avoid lite salad dressings, as they have more carbohydrates. Watch prepared salad dressing for added sugar. Fats are fabulous because they taste good and make you feel full. Dr. Westman says that you can either feel full by stretching your stomach or eating fat. Remember, fat is your new fuel, and it is essential for your new lifestyle!

Cream: up to 2 Tbsp. per day, whipping, heavy, light, or sour cream

<u>Mayonnaise</u>: up to 2 Tbsp. per day

<u>Olives</u>: (black or green) up to 6 per day

<u>Avocado</u>: up to ½ per day

<u>Lemon/lime juice</u>: up to 2 tsp per day

<u>Soy sauces</u>: up to 2 Tbsp. per day

<u>Pickles</u>: (dill or no sugar) 2 per day

<u>Snacks</u>: sugar-free jello, pork rinds, beef jerky, deviled eggs, nuts (almonds, walnuts, pecans)

<u>Sugar Cravings</u>: As your body adjusts, you may crave the sweet stuff...but worry not, this will pass. The less you eat, the sooner the cravings will stop! If it is uncontrollable, have a diet soda or sugar-free jello with whipped cream.

<u>Bouillon</u>: When your body converts from burning carbohydrates for fuel and adapts to burning fat, you may feel a little tired, have a head or body ache, lack focus, or have flu-like symptoms. The symptoms are usually mild, and don't last long. Drink beef or chicken broth 1-3 times a day, unless you have high blood pressure or heart failure. Your energy levels will soon be back. Many people enjoy the broth and continue drinking it!

Just like an alcoholic craves booze, a carboholic craves sugar. And complex carbs are just chains of sugar that are easily converted to sugar, starting with the saliva in your mouth! For weight loss and to eliminate cravings, the only carbs recommended are the very nutritious fiber-rich vegetables on the list.

AVOID: white sugar, brown sugar, honey, maple syrup, molasses, corn syrup, beer, milk (contains lactose), flavored yogurt, fruit juice, and fruit (small portions of berries excluded). Also...grains, whole grains, rice, cereal, flour, bread, pasta, muffins, bagels, crackers, beans, corn, peas, potatoes, canned soups, dairy substitutes, ketchup, sweet relish...BEWARE of "fat-free" or "lite" diet products, and hidden sugar in food like coleslaw. (Confession: I haven't quite given up ketchup yet.) Read labels, and ask the chef in restaurants. You may be surprised about products that are labeled, "Great for Low-Carb Diets"! (They usually aren't).

I am frequently asked about including alcohol in a healthy diet. Needless to say, the best thing for you to drink is water. Some people find that drinking alcohol keeps them from losing weight or messes with blood sugar. If you really enjoy a drink or two, and it isn't interfering with your life, either physically, spiritually, or emotionally, experiment and see how you do with it. Red wine is a good low carb choice, beer is not (Unless it is specifically a low carb beer).

Red wines:

Merlot: 3.7 carbs

Pinot Noir: 3.4 carbs

Cabernet: 3.8 carbs

White wines:

Chardonnay: 3.7 carbs

Pinot Grigio: 3.2 carbs

Riesling: 5.5 carbs

Champagne/Sparking whites: 1.5 carbs

Eat (high fat low carb) when you are hungry, and stop eating when you are full! If you are *not* hungry, you DO NOT HAVE TO EAT!!! Listen to your body (unless it tells you to eat more carbs). Eating less carbs will reduce your appetite. Eating full fat will keep you full! Enjoy the freedom.

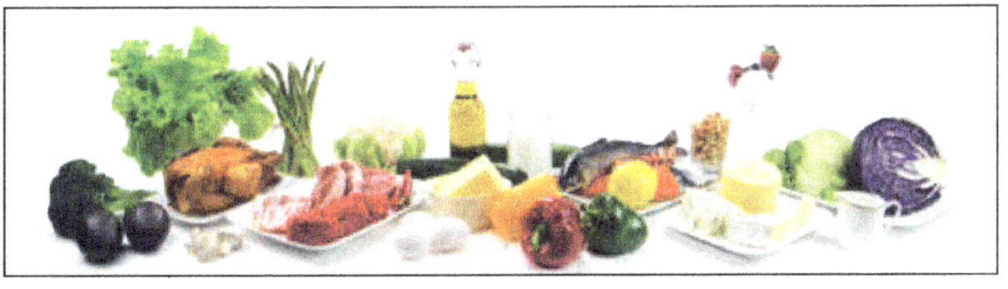

Meal Planning

Finding out that you can abstain from fast-acting, blood sugar hijacking, carbohydrates makes food choices simple and meal planning a snap. One of the most frequently asked questions after people hear that I don't eat carbs, is "What *do* you eat?" Because our Standard American Diet (SAD) is FILLED with many empty fattening carbohydrates, people can't imagine meal planning without them.

Some people are better at planning than others, it seems to come naturally. (Not to me!) But planning ahead makes life a whole lot easier when it comes to meals. When you have made the decision to eat low carb, some planning will help determine the success of your decision.

There's a certain amount of relief once a decision has been made, in other areas as well as what we are going to eat. Whether it's a budget to follow, a trip to take, a career or educational endeavor, the angst of trying to decide is much more stressful than actually doing it. And experts in the field of behavioral change say it is often times better to (like the Nike slogan) "just do it", than to try to gradually make the change. Gradual makes it hard to gain momentum.

Before you start, take a look at the food list you've made. This will spark ideas for meals and snacks for your first week. Having the decision made ahead of time removes the stress of trying to decide when you're hungry! If you're a detailed planner, make a list of recipes and exactly what you will eat. You will be amazed that in no time at all (with consistency) low carb shopping, cooking, and eating will be second nature.

"We can arrange better expectations and better circumstances beginning with the fact that we need not be who we are now; we can be better."
Charles C. Harpe

Clean the Pantry!!! Quite a few of usual pantry items are not an option for the low carb lifestyle. Carbs are very tempting when they are readily available. Your pantry may be in need of a makeover, making it easier to navigate. Go through each shelf, and made sure it contains nothing to tempt you, to dip your hand in and just grab a few... (for example Wheat Thins) Pretty easy to dip into. Carb snacking will annihilate your resolve, perhaps triggering a carbohydrate binge! If there are members of your family who don't want to adopt your new plan, at least make yourself a shelf. Put canned goods, containers of nuts and sugar-free candy for treats where they're easy to reach. That way when you are in the mood for a snack you have something handy.

It is helpful that the government requires food producers to put nutrition labels on our food. Don't be deceived in thinking these numbers are perfectly accurate, though. There is a margin of error that they deem perfectly acceptable. In her blog, nutritionist Tamara Duker Freuman states that the numbers can be off by 20% either way. She goes on to say "The best guidance I can offer is to minimize the number of foods in your diet that even *have* a nutrition label; eating more whole, unpackaged, minimally-processed foods is likely to bump up the quality of your diet."

After your pantry make-over, clean out the refrigerator! Your frig will be your best friend in your quest to eat low carb, if you stock it with great high-fat choices and easy to prepare meals. Buy unsweetened coconut milk, almond milk, and always have eggs on hand for an easy protein-filled breakfast.

Meal Planning for Busy People...or "I Hate to Cook!"

Breakfast is easy if you like eggs. I make omelets on weekends, and quick scrambled during the week, adding different meats and cheeses. Cooking your bacon or sausage up ahead is helpful, or using pre-cooked meats like salami or pepperoni. Buy pre-shredded cheese for convenience. Reheating the leftovers from last night's dinner is one of the easiest ways to prepare a nutritious breakfast, it probably has a good serving of protein. Protein is important for getting your body off to a good start, but if you are rushed it is tempting to leave it out. (Hurried people skip breakfast or snag a bagel or bowl of cereal!) I make extra at dinner so that I have enough for breakfast and/or lunch the next day. I also make extra vegetables when I'm cooking them. They can be put in breakfast scramble or omelet. Dairy products such as Greek yogurt, ricotta cheese, or cottage cheese can be combined with berries, nuts or flax seed to make a quick breakfast. Add some cream in your coffee if you like but avoid sweetened creamers.

I also add some veggies, or a small glass of V-8. A protein shake or a green vegetable smoothie are great options.

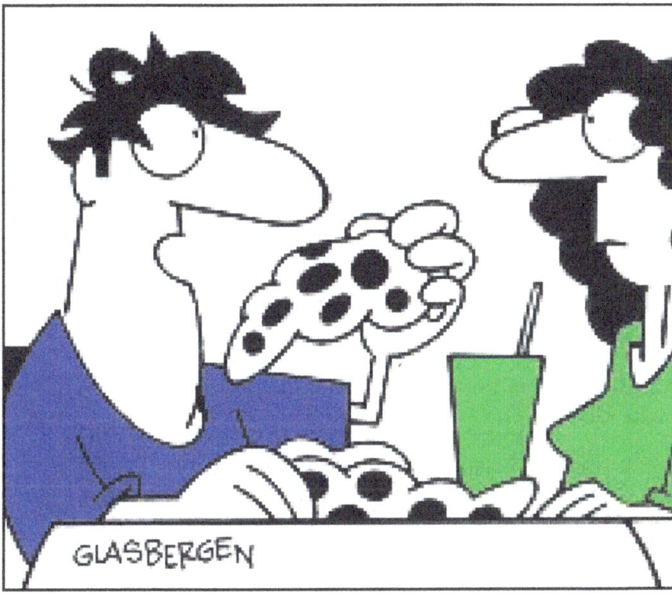

"The sauce has tomatoes and oregano. The crust is basically a big crouton. Technically, pizza is a salad!"

Lunches include great ideas like egg-salad (if I didn't have eggs for breakfast), tuna salad, sliced turkey, chicken, or beef (we like peppered turkey and beef) and various cheeses rolled in a low carb tortilla or lettuce. Cheese or peanut butter with celery is a great crunchy option, and jicama is also a good crunch. It can help make the transition from chips to veggies easier for those crunch addicts. Same as in breakfast, if you don't have time for vegetables a small glass of V8 rounds it out.

On the go breakfast or lunches can include scooping your eggs/meat/cheese/lettuce/condiments into a low carb tortilla, wrap in foil and you're out the door!

Go crazy at dinner. Salmon, other fish or shellfish, steak, burgers, chicken, pork chops or roasts...and add a vegetable and a salad! You will, in time, lose the feeling that you have to add starchy foods to your meal. Hang tough; resist the thought that you *need* potatoes, rice, pasta, bread, etc. Even guests at my home are thrilled to see that they don't have to eat starch and sugar just to be nice or because they don't want to offend the hostess. This is especially true at parties. Christmas 2013 was my first attempt at hosting and catering a low-carb wine and jazz party. It was a huge success! You will find the recipes in the recipe section to get started entertaining low carb. Your guests will thank you.

Growth demands a temporary surrender of security. It may mean giving up familiar but limiting patterns, safe but unrewarding work, values no longer believed in, and relationships that have lost their meaning.
John C. Maxwell

CHAPTER 13

The Family Chef
Tim Ferch

When my sister was diagnosed with Type 1 diabetes, I flew into a rage. How could this happen to me? Anger...resentment... denial...well, just a few of my many emotions. What could this mean? She wouldn't be eating my fabulous stuffing, mashed potatoes, and most of all my amazing gravy. This simply could not be happening to me. No more wonderful spaghetti, stroganoff or goulash. And what about my breakfast frittata, filled with potatoes? I figured my world was basically over. This left me with one basic choice since I have been doing a large portion of our family's cooking for the last few years.

I needed to look into my mirror, address my semi-narcissistic self-absorbed self with my chubby belly and go with the reality that I needed to begin thinking in terms of low carb recipes that could give all the emotional satisfaction of a plate full of carbs without the health consequences. (Let me say right here and now that my gut is gone thanks to my new attitude and personal food choices.)

I began thinking about ideas and how to use pioneering concepts. Thinking of Asian, I began with cauliflower rice. If chopped correctly, it has the same consistency, flavor, and texture as actual rice. Combine this with flavors and ingredients of your favorite stir fry and you will have a wonderful meal. Keep being creative with your other ingredients and flavor techniques.

On to Italian. Even though it is a well-known fact that Italians are the best lovers…let's just imagine that your Italian lover had a flat stomach with well-defined abs. *That* would be the result of a LCHF diet. Imagine, ladies, all the passion of your Italian Stallion without the hug with the gut.

I find it personally painful to see my sister, by all appearances, have to treat food as a necessary evil. Meals have always been a huge part of our family fun. From Grandma's buffets to feed endless cowboys at cattle-working events like branding, to holidays with bottomless bowls of mashed potatoes and at least 5 kinds of pie. During the process of learning to cook low carb, it became a challenge and even a lot of fun to come up with appetizing alternatives to our former carbohydrate consuming calendar. Sadly, our Grandma ended up with type 2 diabetes and it became her struggle too. I can see now that it's better for our family to eat a lower carb fare, and as a matter of fact it can still involve great eating.

When I decided spend some time in Scottsdale, little did I know, my diet would change forever too. With both my sister and her husband being Type 1 diabetics, my carb filled diet was about to change. While thinking that a low carb diet was a *necessity* for diabetics I had no idea of the benefits it would bring to me, the average person. I changed out of necessity to eat with the family and began to realize a consistent energy level without the ups and downs of the carb binge. You know... big meal followed by a long nap, or if there wasn't a couch handy, a struggle to stay awake. Even though I am genetically predisposed to having a tall, lanky frame, when I approached fifty I turned sideways in the mirror and suddenly realized that I looked like a snake that had swallowed a tennis ball. The gut was unacceptable.

I had no idea that a consistent low carb diet over the following four months would melt away my tummy back to the flat condition reminiscent of my twenties. I also have one confession...In the middle of that four months I took a trip back to Montana. During that trip I decided to fix my amazing Mexican style breakfast complete with refried beans, Spanish rice, tortillas and trimmings. That evening we enjoyed a couple bowls of chili with beans. Needless to say a carb binge fit for a king. A small bout with IBS followed by a lethargic two day recovery period made me run back to eating low carb, and along with it came consistent energy that I have been enjoying ever since. I simply had no idea what a shock to the system a barrage of carb/sugar would do to my system after the consistency of a healthy diet. I don't plan to make that mistake again.

While it is possible to eat LCHF and spend little to no time in the kitchen, some of us really enjoy cooking. And for those who do, here are a few of our family's favorite recipes.

STARTER

Ferch's Famous Shrimp Cocktail

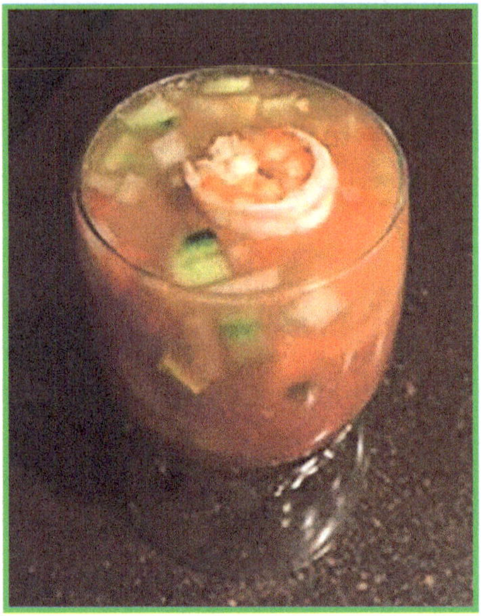

I ended up drunk on my 22nd birthday in Mexico, (that was before rehab) and vaguely remembered eating this amazing dish. About 5 years later, my parents and I went to Nogales, where I walked from store to store, describing the place to anyone who could or couldn't speak English. I finally found a girl at a cosmetic store and she said, "Oh yeah, it's about two blocks south of here." My taste buds led me back to exactly what I remembered. An outdoor stand with bar stools, a countertop, and a little back room and poles that held up an awning. I found it, watched the chef, came home and messed with it till it matched the authentic Mexican flavor. I serve these at any event, Super bowl parties, Christmas Eve, etc. Or a movie-night snack. It's a great starter or even a light meal.

Ingredients

1 lb. uncooked small shrimp (41-60 count)
½ lb small scallops (optional)
1 medium yellow onion
1 English cucumber
4 medium ripe tomatoes
6 limes
2 cans Spicy V8

Instructions

1. Cook seafood in 3 c. boiling water. 3-4 minutes till done, do not overcook. Chill.
2. Juice limes, and add juice and V8 to seafood. Chill.
3. Dice onion, cucumber and tomatoes very small.
4. Divide chopped vegetables and seafood evenly in 4-6 cocktail glasses. Top off with remaining liquid, add salt, lime juice or hot sauce to taste. I prefer Red Hot which is made with a variety of cayenne peppers to Tabasco.

MAIN COURSES
Caper Chicken by Nikos Ligidakis

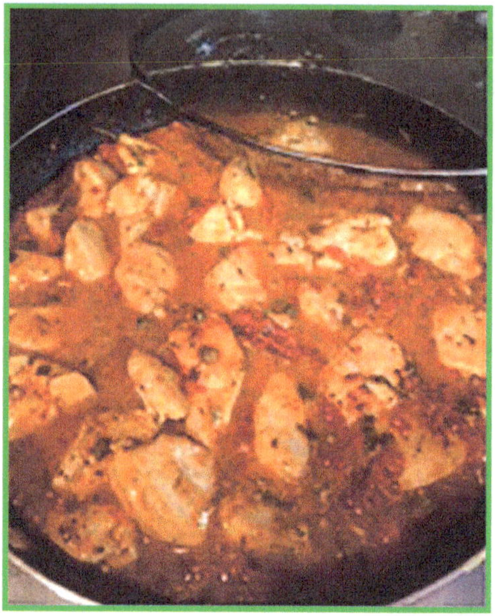

This AMAZING recipe was an INSTANT success. Discovered quite by accident, when my brother-in-law decided to try and cook for about 100 of my sister's closest friends at her 50th birthday party. When he called our friend Nick (Amazing Chef turned Book Publisher and the Publisher of this book), Nick sensed that he was in over his head and offered to do the cooking. This recipe is fondly called "Nick's Chicken" and squeals of delight are heard from everyone when we're having it for dinner!

Ingredients

Olive oil
Chicken breasts cut in quarters
4 Chopped Roma tomatoes
4 tbsp. capers (found in the olive section of most grocery stores)
½ c. Sun-dried tomatoes cut in large pieces
1 tbsp. chopped garlic
*Sliced zucchini is optional
1 c. white wine
Black pepper to taste
2 tbsp. basil
2 tbsp. parsley
1 tbsp. oregano
1 tbsp. thyme
1 tbsp. rosemary

Instructions

1. Brown chicken pieces in olive oil.
2. Add the rest of the ingredients and simmer uncovered for 45 minutes.

Pizza

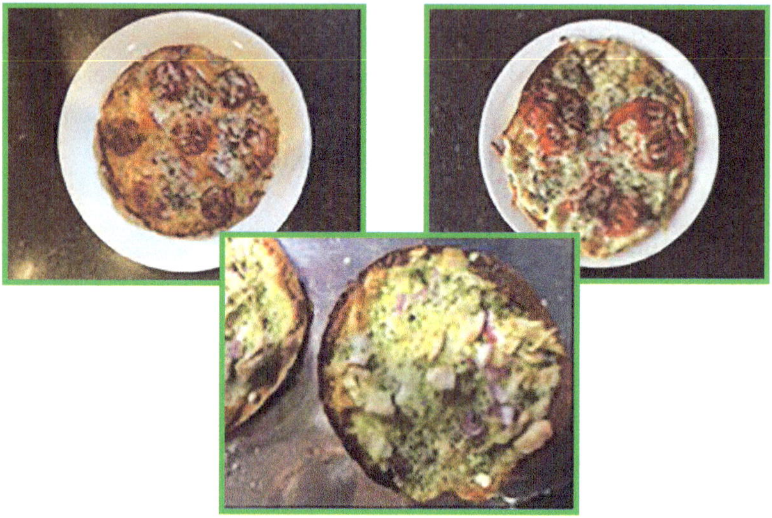

Pizza variations are endless, only limited by your imagination and personal tastes. The trick to making the crust crispy enough with a low carb tortilla takes a few extra minutes, but worth the time if you want to pick it up and eat it like the real thing.

Ingredients
Low carb tortillas
Melted butter
Shredded mozzarella cheese

Instructions

1. Brush tortillas with butter.
2. Bake in 425 degree oven till crispy.
3. Add a thin layer of cheese and bake till melted. This keeps the sauce from soaking in and crust crispy plus tastes great!
4. Add sauce, toppings, bake, and serve!

Topping Favorites:

1. Marinara sauce
2. Thin sliced tomatoes
3. Pepperoni
4. Sausage
5. Shredded cheese of any kind
6. Ground Parmesan

Or…

1. Pesto as the sauce
2. Chicken Pieces
3. Red onion

Or…

1. Alfredo as the sauce
2. Shrimp
3. Mushrooms
4. Artichoke hearts

Sprinkle Italian Blend Seasoning on the top
Bake at 400 for 20 min or until lightly browned

Cheesy Chicken stuffed Poblano Peppers

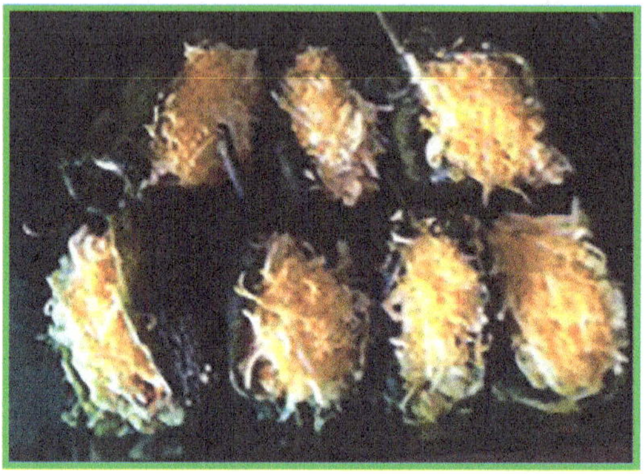

This one is for those who don't mind a little time in the kitchen. A great "company dinner" with a southwestern flair you can make ahead of time!

Ingredients

Roasted Poblano Peppers (Anaheim peppers can substitute/ may be hotter)
3 c. Chicken Chunks
8 oz. Softened Cream Cheese
½ c. Grated Pepper Jack Cheese
½ c. Sour Cream
1 4 oz. can Chopped Green Chilies
Salt & Pepper to Taste
¾ c. Grated Cheddar Cheese

Instructions

1. Rub peppers with olive oil and roast in hot (400 degrees) oven, turning often till all sides are toasty.
2. Put hot peppers into a paper bag and seal, to steam. When cooled enough to touch, gently peel outer thin skin from peppers and slice one side, remove seeds.
3. Mix chicken, softened cream cheese, pepper jack cheese, sour cream, green chilies, and salt and pepper in medium sauce pan.
4. Heat mixture and stuff peppers.
5. Top with grated cheddar cheese and bake for 20 minutes at 350 degrees.

Shepherd's Pie with Cauliflower Crust

This is an amazing one dish meal…courtesy of my sister's friend Andrea. Perfect if you need something to pull out of the oven and put on the table. Friends sharing low carb makes for excellent variation in meals. Check out the cookbook Low-Carbing Among Friends. Available at www.amongfriends.us.

Ingredients

Meat mixture

1 lb. mild pork sausage
2 lb. hamburger
1 medium carrot, chopped
1 medium onion chopped
1 stalk celery, chopped
2 cloves garlic, chopped
½ c. chopped parsley

8 oz. chopped French green beans
1 tsp. rosemary
1 bay leaf
Salt and pepper
Beef stock, as needed

Cauliflower Topping

Head of cauliflower
½ c. sour cream
4 tbsp. butter
½ c. cheddar cheese, shredded
¼ c. parmesan cheese
8 oz. Gouda cheese, shredded
1 tsp. garlic powder
Salt & Pepper to taste
1 tsp. chicken bouillon

Instructions

1. Pre-heat oven to 350 degrees
2. Steam the cauliflower until very soft. Drain well.
3. While the cauliflower is still very warm, blend it in a food processor, adding all the cauliflower topping ingredients except the Gouda cheese. Blend until very smooth. Set aside.
4. Brown the sausage and hamburger.
5. Add the vegetables and the rest of the meat mixture ingredients. Simmer for 20 more minutes.
6. In a deep, oven-safe casserole dish, layer the Meat Mixture at the bottom.
7. Cover with the Cauliflower Topping.
8. Sprinkle the shredded Gouda on top.

Bake about 30 minutes until the meat mixture is bubbly and the cheese gets a little brown and crusty.

Salmon Fillets with Avocado Cucumber and Dill Salsa

Ingredients

1 med. European cucumber, cut into ½ inch pieces
2 tbsp. finely chopped dill
2 tbsp. olive oil
2 tbsp. rice wine vinegar
1 tbsp. fresh lemon juice
½ tsp. salt
½ tsp. Splenda or Stevia
1 ripe small avocado, peeled, pitted, and cut into ¼ inch pieces
1 tbsp. fresh lemon juice
1 tbsp. finely chopped fresh dill

Instructions

1. Combine all the salsa ingredients in a medium mixing bowl and taste for seasoning. Set aside.
2. Sprinkle salmon fillets evenly with the lemon juice and chopped dill.
3. Grill on BBQ. Medium heat.
4. Top with salsa, garnish with lemon slices and fresh dill sprigs. Serve immediately.

Salsa can be prepared up to 4 hours ahead and refrigerated. Salsa good on cold salmon as well.

Beer Brats

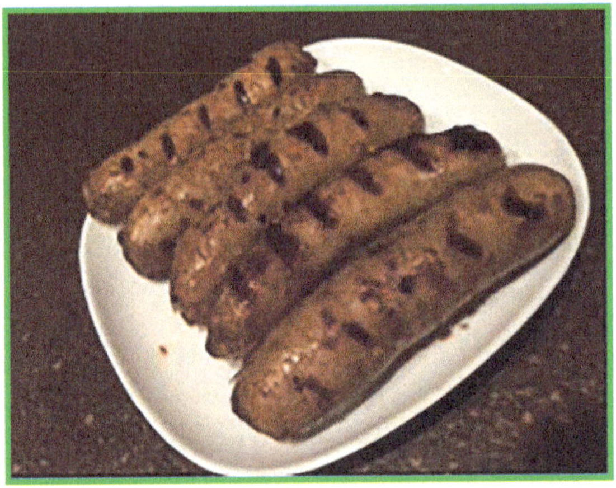

Ingredients
10 bratwurst
2 cans beer
2 tbsp. red pepper flakes
1 large onion, diced
1 tbsp. chopped fresh garlic or 1 tsp garlic powder
1 tsp salt
½ tsp. ground black pepper

Instructions

1. Combine all ingredients except brats, bring to a boil.
2. Add brats and add water till they're covered.
3. Simmer 12-15 minutes.
4. Remove brats and send them out to the BBQ with designated grill person.

Green Chile Pork

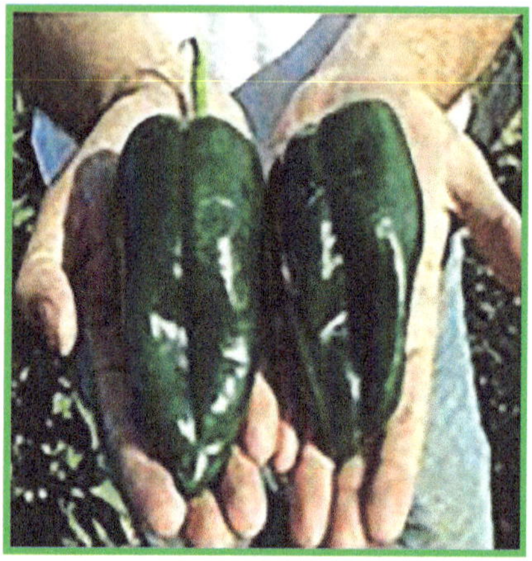

Poblano peppers are a mild chili, originating from Puebla, Mexico.

When my sister came home for Christmas, looking forward to treating the family to Green Chili Pork on Christmas Eve, and left her peppers in Arizona, she was really sad! She thought there would never be a Poblano in Montana. However, they are becoming increasingly popular and we discovered them at a small organic grocery chain called Lucky's Market. Christmas Eve was saved!

Ingredients

2 tbsp. olive oil

2 lbs. coarsely cut boneless country-style pork ribs, pork loin roast, or tenderloin

2 c. diced yellow onion

¼ c. minced jalapeno chilies

1 small can minced New Mexico green chilies

¼ c. minced garlic

6 Poblano peppers

1 c. grated pepper jack cheese

Instructions

1. Rub peppers with oil and roast at 425 degrees (hot oven) turning periodically till blackened.
2. Remove from oven and put in paper bag, cool.
3. Peel waxy coating from peppers, remove seeds, and puree in food processor. Set aside.
4. Season pork with salt and pepper.
5. Heat the oil. When hot, add pork, onions, jalapeno, New Mexico green chilies, and garlic.
6. Roast pork till internal temperature is 160 degrees, followed by a three minute rest. Cut into cubes.
7. Add the Poblano puree to meat, and simmer for 45 min. Season to taste with salt and pepper. Top with grated cheese.

Alexa's Seasoned Burgers

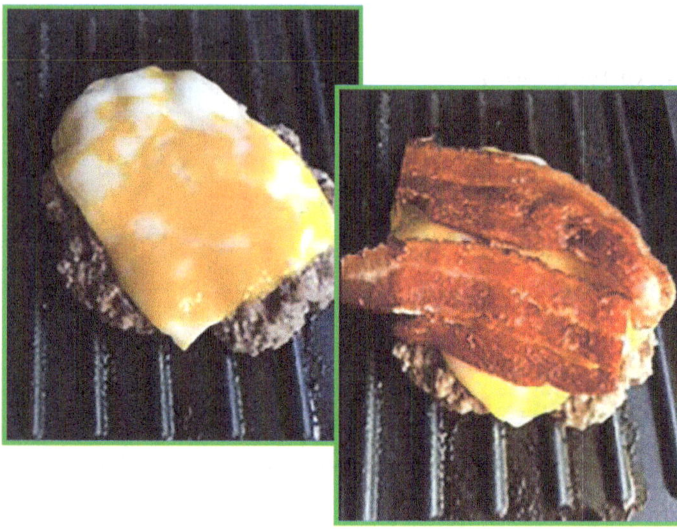

Burgers are an all-time American Favorite, and the way my niece Alexa seasons the meat is always good! It is up to you if you prefer grass-fed, organic, etc. And bacon always makes it better.

Ingredients
1 lb. ground beef
1 tsp. minced garlic
1 tbsp. Worcestershire Sauce
1 tsp. onion powder
1 tsp. salt
½ tsp. black pepper
(optional cayenne pepper to taste)
(optional add bacon bits to the meat mixture)

Instructions
Mash seasonings with ground beef and send outside to the designated grill person. We use a George Forman inside for small crowds.

Unforgettable Burger Option

(My roommate, Dave, was still talking about this one the next morning)

1. Make a batch of the Ultimate Gravy (page 201).
2. Cook burgers.
3. Serve over riced cauliflower cooked with a few peas and onions.

Pork Tenderloin with Apples & Bacon

We made this for a family dinner, I was thinking my dad, a Montana Meat-Eating Cowboy would think it was too fluffy with the apples. He surprised me though, and said it was the best pork roast he had ever eaten. Yep, made it into the "make it again" recipe category!

Ingredients

1 ½ lb. pork tenderloin
3 slices bacon
½ c. apple cider vinegar
½ c. water
¼ c. Splenda or Stevia to taste
1 small Jonathan apple, peeled and cut into small pieces

Instructions

1. Fry bacon, remove, set aside to cool and crumble.
2. Cook tenderloin in bacon fat. (I braise it and stick it in the oven)
3. Add water, sugar, and vinegar to pork drippings and bring to a boil. 4. Add apple pieces and cook to soften/reduce liquid.

Add crumbled bacon and pour over pork slices.

Meat Balls

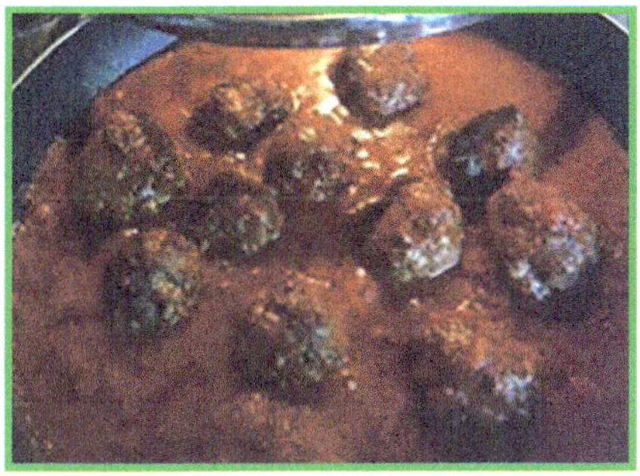

Ingredients

1 lb. ground beef
1/3 lb. breakfast sausage
1/3 c. Italian bread crumbs
1 egg
1 Tbsp. Worcestershire Sauce
¼ c. almond milk, unsweetened
¾ tsp. Italian Blend Seasoning
¼ tsp. cayenne pepper
¼ tsp. salt
1/3 c. grated parmesan cheese
1 tsp. fresh minced garlic

Instructions

1. Mix all ingredients together
2. Roll into 1 ½ inch balls
3. Bake approx. 30 minutes till done
4. Serve with Marinara sauce or sauce of choice and vegi-noodles.

Caesar Pork Chops

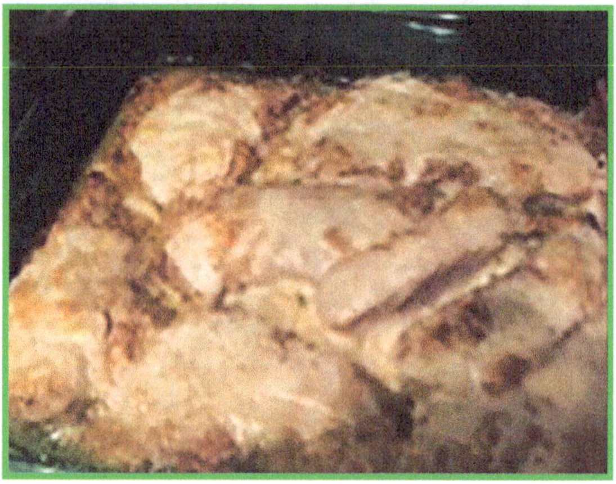

Ingredients

½ c almond flour

½ tsp. Italian seasoning

½ c Caesar salad dressing

4 bone-in pork chops, ½ inch thick

½ c ground parmesan cheese

1 c. mozzarella cheese, shredded

Instructions

1. Preheat oven to 375 degrees
2. Put almond flour in shallow dish (spray with PAM or olive oil)
3. Mix Caesar dressing, Italian seasoning, and parmesan cheese and put in another shallow dish.
4. Dip pork chops in dressing mixture, and then almond flour
5. Arrange in baking dish
6. Bake 25 minutes
7. Top with shredded mozzarella and bake 10-15 minutes until pork is no longer pink in the center.

Brussels Sprouts with Shallots

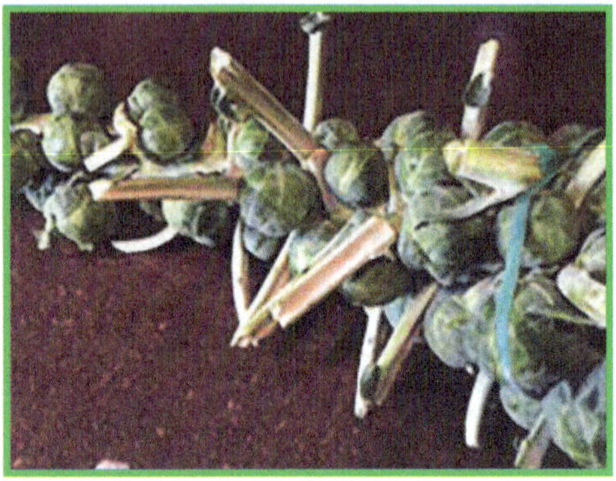

Since opening my mind to the possibility of eating a wider variety of green vegetables, I came across this "to die for" recipe when my friend Sheryl brought it to Thanksgiving Dinner. I have tried many others since but none compare to the salty/sweet/tangy version of this one. Adapted to low carb from an Epicurious Magazine version.

Ingredients

6 tbsp. Butter
½ lb. Shallots, chopped or sliced
Salt & Pepper
2 tbsp. apple cider vinegar
1 tbsp. Splenda
1 ½ lb. Brussels sprouts, halved lengthwise & trimmed
3 tbsp. Extra Virgin Olive Oil
1 c. water

Instructions

1. Melt butter in skillet over medium heat. Add shallots, salt and pepper
2. Sauté till golden brown, about 6 minutes
3. Add vinegar and Splenda, stir till golden (1-3 minutes) and set aside
4. Heat oil in large skillet, add sprouts and sprinkle with salt and pepper
5. Sauté until brown at edges, 6 minutes.
6. Add 1 c. water and 3 tbsp. butter.
7. Sauté until most of the water evaporates, about 5 minutes.
8. Add shallots back to the pan, season with salt and pepper.

Garlic Roasted Brussels Sprouts

Ingredients

1 lb. Brussels sprouts
2 cloves minced garlic
1 tsp. cayenne pepper
4 Tbsp. olive oil
2 tsp. fresh lemon juice

Instructions

1. Boil Brussels sprouts for 2-3 minutes
2. Transfer to baking pan
3. Mix olive oil, cayenne pepper and lemon juice
4. Drizzle over sprouts
5. Bake, shaking occasionally until crispy on the outside and tender on the inside. Squeeze fresh lime to taste when serving.

Butternut Squash Bisque

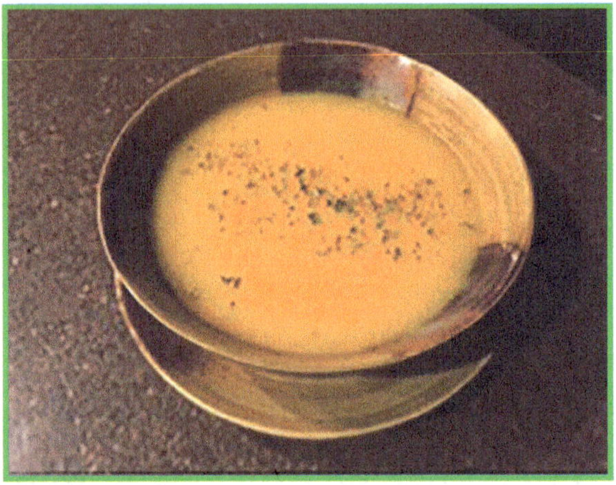

This delicious bisque is a perfect starter for a dinner party on a fall or winter evening. I serve it with ribs or grilled chicken as a meal. Perfectly good the next day which makes it ideal to make ahead and reheat. You can also freeze it.

Ingredients

6 c. cubed Butternut Squash

¼ c. finely chopped Yellow Onion

4 c. Chicken Broth

Salt/Pepper

Cayenne Pepper or Nutmeg

Instructions

1. Bring broth to a boil and add squash (cut into ½ inch cubes)
2. Add chopped onion
3. Simmer over low heat 45-50 minutes or until squash cubes mash easily.
4. Cool slightly and puree in blender or food processor till smooth
5. Add pinch of cayenne and/or nutmeg and salt and pepper to taste.
6. Garnish with parsley if desired.

Cayenne Pepper or Nutmeg

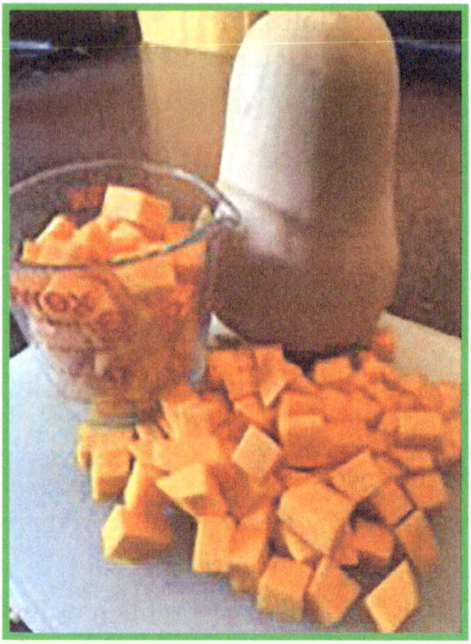

Instructions

1. Bring broth to a boil and add squash (cut into ½ inch cubes)
2. Add chopped onion
3. Simmer over low heat 45-50 minutes or until squash cubes mash easily.
4. Cool slightly and puree in blender or food processor till smooth
5. Add pinch of cayenne and/or nutmeg and salt and pepper to taste.
6. Garnish with parsley if desired.

Zucchini & Yellow Squash Medley

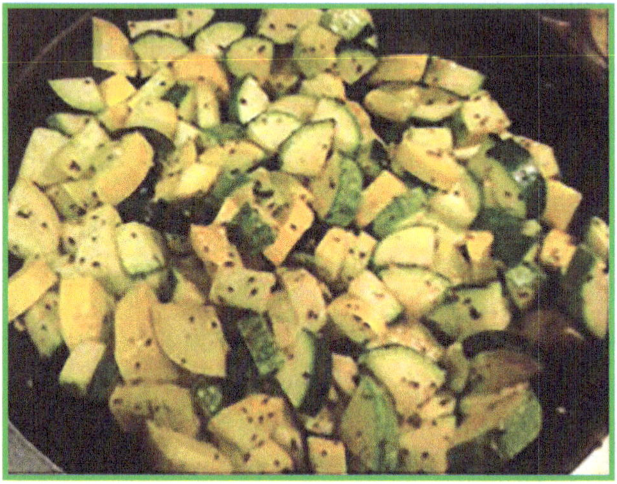

I remember the first year my grandma planted zucchini. It was a bumper crop, and as kids we had to eat EVERYTHING zucchini. Fried, poached, boiled in soup, and even in brownies. She thought they were so moist. We thought they tasted terrible. By now our taste buds are more sophisticated and have adapted to zucchini… but definitely like it al dente with garlic and basil and not cooked to death like Grandma used to do!

Ingredients

1 ½ c. yellow squash

1 ½ c. zucchini

2 tbsp. olive oil

1 tsp. chopped garlic

3 tbsp. dried basil

1 tsp. salt

½ tsp. fresh ground pepper

Instructions

1. Heat olive oil in medium skillet
2. Add squash and spices Sautee until al dente

"Riced" Cauliflower

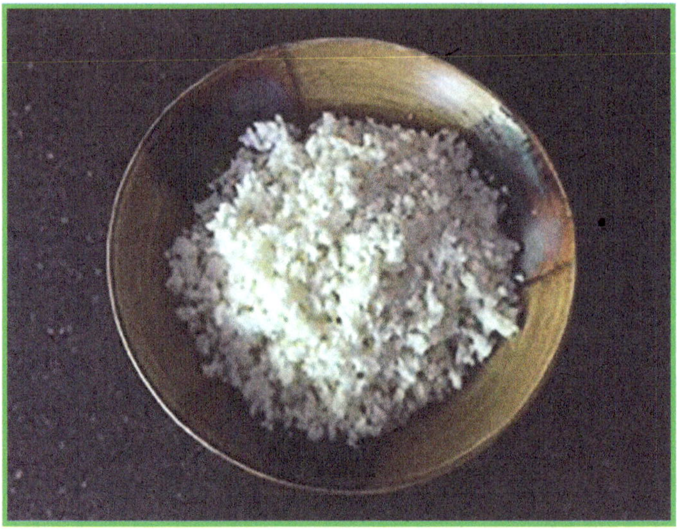

Very useful substitute for rice. You can make anything out of riced cauliflower when you would normally use rice. It's great as a simple side with garlic/onion/butter/salt or as an ingredient in fried rice, side dish for stir-fry, Spanish rice, you get the picture.

Ingredients

Cauliflower

Olive Oil

Optional: Garlic, Onion, Salt & Pepper to taste.

Instructions

Thoroughly wash cauliflower and cut into pieces

Fill food processor ½ full (at the most) and pulse until cauliflower is the size of rice kernels. If you fill the processor too full the bottom will become pureed and the top will stay too chunky.

Remove any chunks and set aside for next batch.

Heat olive oil and desired spices in large frying pan, toss in cauliflower and sauté for 4-6 minutes until softened. Remove from heat and serve or add spices. Can be substituted in any recipe calling for rice.

Cauliflower Posing as Mashed Potatoes

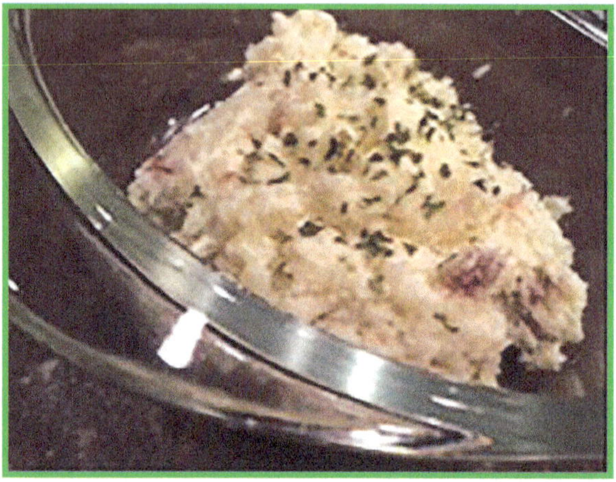

I really didn't think it was possible to pull this one off. I have tasted the "faux-tatoes" in other settings and didn't like them so much. But this one works like a dream come true! Yummm.

Ingredients

1 head of cauliflower
2 c. chicken broth
1 tsp. minced garlic
(optional)peelings of 2 red potatoes
¼ c. sour cream
4 oz. softened cream cheese
1 tsp. garlic powder
1 tsp. onion powder
ranch dressing (optional)
salt & pepper
¼ c. softened butter

Instructions

1. Bring chicken broth and garlic to a boil, add cauliflower cut into chunks
2. Boil till softened (approximately 20 minutes) (Last 5 minutes add potato peelings)
3. Drain liquid
4. Puree cooked cauliflower in food processor
5. Add sour cream, cream cheese, garlic powder, onion powder, ranch dressing, salt & pepper and butter
6. Cream together
7. Garnish with parsley flakes if desired
8. Serve immediately or set over pan of hot water to keep warm

Making Gravy

Dry Substitutes

DRY Ingredient	Amount	Calories	Carbohydrates	Fiber	Net Carbs	Protein
Almond Flour	1 Tbsp	40	1	1	0	6
Arrowroot Flour	1 tsp	19	4.7	0	4.7	0.01
Chia Seed	1 Tbsp	50	4	4	0	2
Coconut Flour	1 Tbsp	30	2	1	1	1
Cornstarch	.5 Tbsp	15	3.9	0.03	3.9	0.01
Flax Seed Meal	1 Tbsp	30	0	2	0	2
Tapioca Pearls	1 Tbsp	14	4	0	4	0
Wheat Flour	1 Tbsp	31	6.2	0.2	6	1.03

I found this chart interesting when it comes to thickening agents. As previously stated…I am a gravy guy. And Dr. Hilts agrees with me on this!

Ultimate Gravy

Ingredients

6 green onions
2 c. beef or chicken stock
½ tsp. Lawry's or Johnny's Seasoning
½ tsp. pepper
1 tbsp. cornstarch
2 tbsp. additional thickener of choice
1 clove garlic
2 tbsp. butter

Instructions

1. Chop onions, sauté the white part of the onion in a large fry pan in butter
2. Dissolve the thickening agent in in ½ c. of the stock, add a sprinkle of Lawry's or Johnny's Seasoning, and salt and pepper to taste.
3. Whisk into sautéed onions, add remaining stock, and lightly boil until thickened.
4. Garnish with the chopped green part of onions.

Cheesy Cauliflower Bake

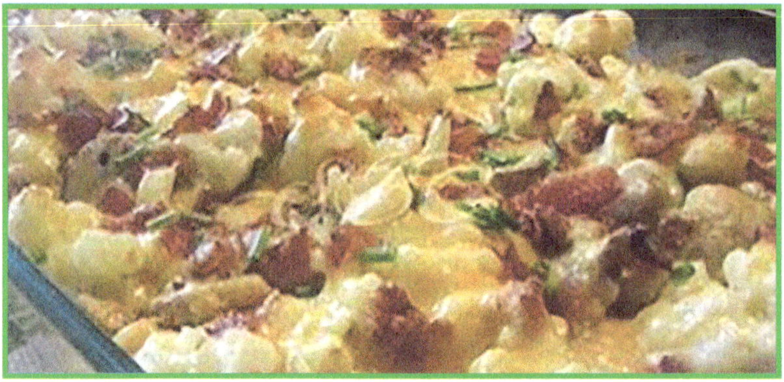

This is a great low carb alternative to a casserole, either scalloped potatoes or macaroni and cheese. Again, borrowed from our friend, Andrea. Simple and delicious!

Ingredients

1 head cauliflower

sautéed diced yellow onion (optional)

1 c. grated colby-jack cheese or cheddar

1 c. bacon bits

2 tbsp. butter

Instructions

1. Steam cauliflower pieces till al dente
2. Spread in baking dish
3. Sautee onion in butter/cook bacon and cut in pieces
4. Scatter onion and bacon bits
5. Cover with cheese
6. Bake in oven at 350 degrees till cheese is melted
7. Garnish with green onion and sour cream

Another Very Useful Side Dish

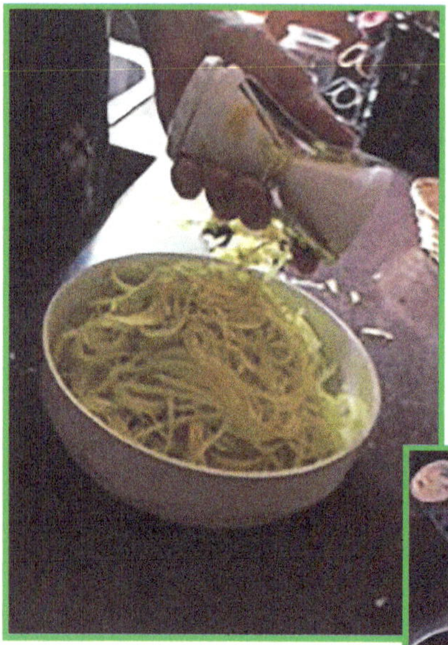

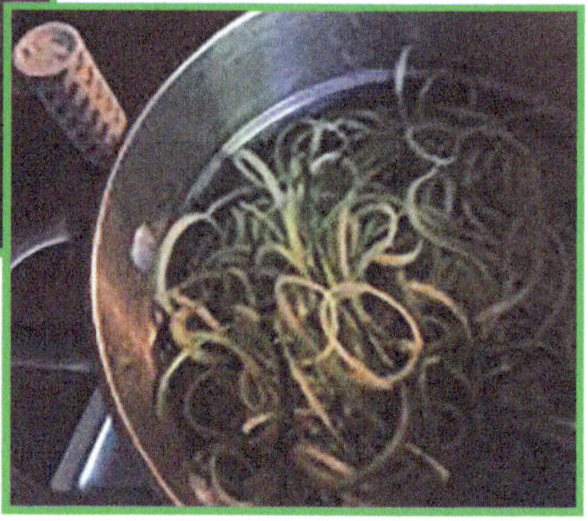

Using a "Veggetti", which I bought at Target in the As Seen on TV section, I make noodles out of zucchini and/or yellow squash. These noodles can be used fresh, with a hot sauce partially cooking them, or you can quick-fry them in a hot pan with olive oil for a minute or two, and then serve immediately.

NOTES

Breakfast & Brunch

Coconut/Blueberry Crepe Filling

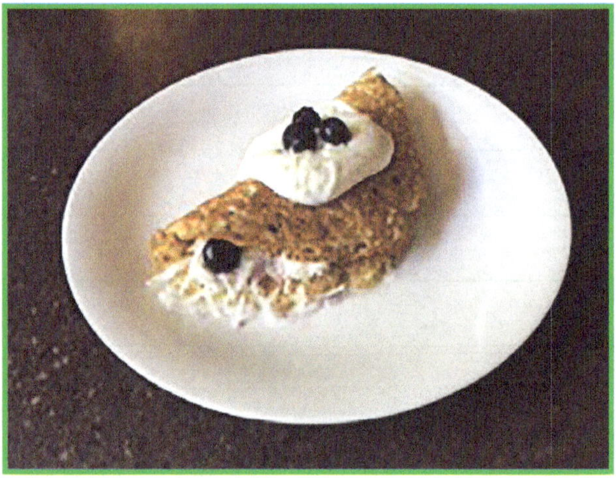

One day when a friend was particularly bummed out about the low-carb life she didn't want to live, I broke out of my usual food routine and came up with this little desert/brunch option. Actually, it's an "anytimeofday" option! A movie at home and crepes. It was an extremely suitable substitute for popcorn!

Ingredients

1 c. cottage cheese

3-4 drops Liquid Stevia

1 tsp. vanilla

¼ c. unsweetened coconut

Blueberries (or raspberries/strawberries)

Whipped cream

Instructions

1. Mix cottage cheese and stevia to desired sweetness
2. Add coconut and blueberries
   Fold crepe and top with sugar-free whipped crème

Crepes

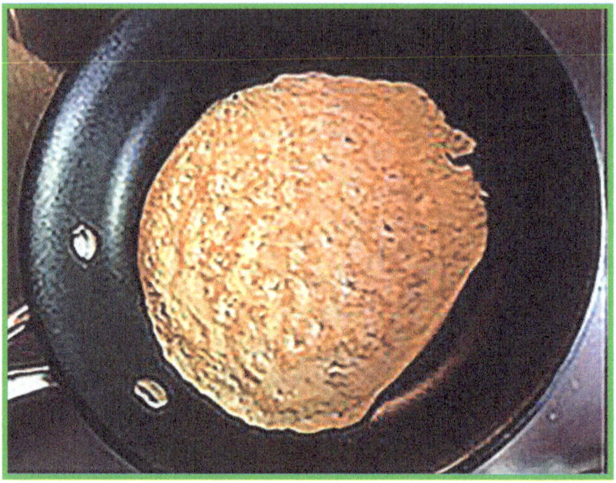

These crepes are a great way to sneak in a little protein on Sunday brunch or can be a healthy desert, depending on the filling. The variations are endless!

Ingredients

4 ounces cream cheese, softened

4 large eggs

3/4 c. almond flour

2 tbsp. flour

1 tbsp. Splenda (or Stevia equivalent)

1/4 cup unsweetened almond milk

Pinch salt

Instructions

1. Combine all ingredients in food processor or blender.
2. Heat non-stick pan on medium heat. Add just enough oil or butter to the pan to lightly coat it. Once hot, pour enough batter to the pan so it is about 5 inches in diameter and swirl into a thin layer that reaches the edges.
3. Cook until edges are cooked and can be loosened with a spatula. Flip and cook on the other side until lightly browned.

Pancakes!!!

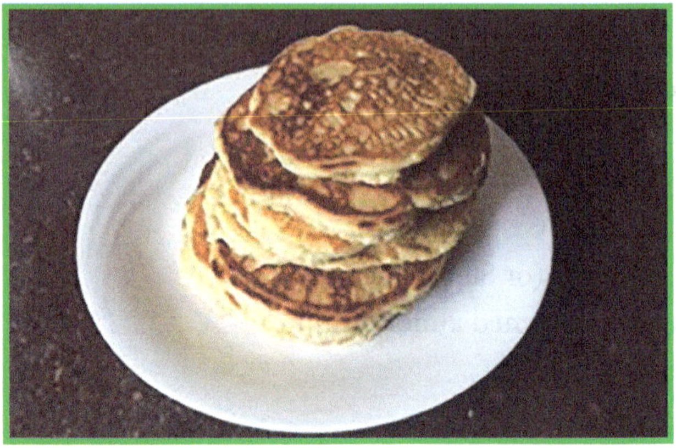

One day I opened a magazine sent out by our insurance company on getting healthy, and found this bad-boy recipe for pancakes…I was ecstatic!!! There are a few things my family misses in the transition from carb-filled meals, and pancakes are one of them. It only took a switch from honey to stevia and the rest is delicious eating history.

Ingredients

3 large eggs
1/3 c pure full fat unsweetened coconut milk
1 tbsp. coconut oil
1 tsp. Stevia or Splenda…can use drops
1 tsp. vanilla
¼ tsp. apple cider vinegar
1 ½ c. almond flour
½ tsp. soda
¼ tsp. salt

Instructions

1. Pre-heat griddle to 350
2. Put the eggs, coconut milk, sweetener, vanilla, and vinegar in blender or food processor.
3. Put soda, salt, and almond flour on top.
4. Blend for a minute, add more coconut milk or a little almond milk if the batter is too thick.
5. Cook 'em and Eat 'em!
   Additionally you can add pecans/blueberries/ unsweetened coconut, walnuts, any number of low carb ingredients for a tasty pancake.

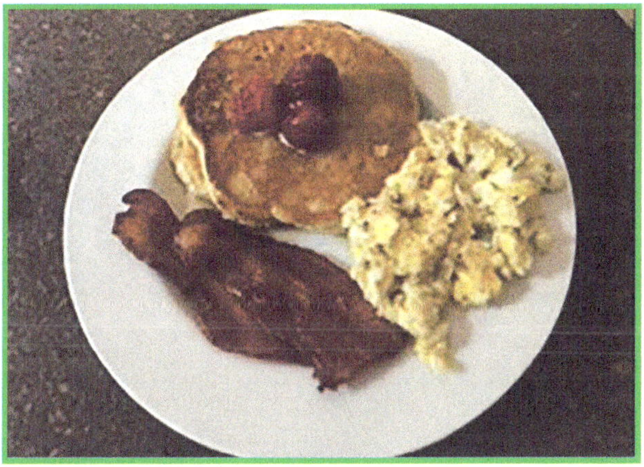

Let's talk about eggs for a minute here…According to Dr. Kaayla Daniel, author of the free eBook The *Fats of Life*, eggs are the perfect food. They have all the vital nutrients we need except Vitamin C. The whites have exceptional protein, and the yolks provide vital fatty acids. She goes on to say if the chickens are raised in a pasture the eggs also provide vitamins A, D, choline, and DHA for nerve function. Yay eggs!

Omelets

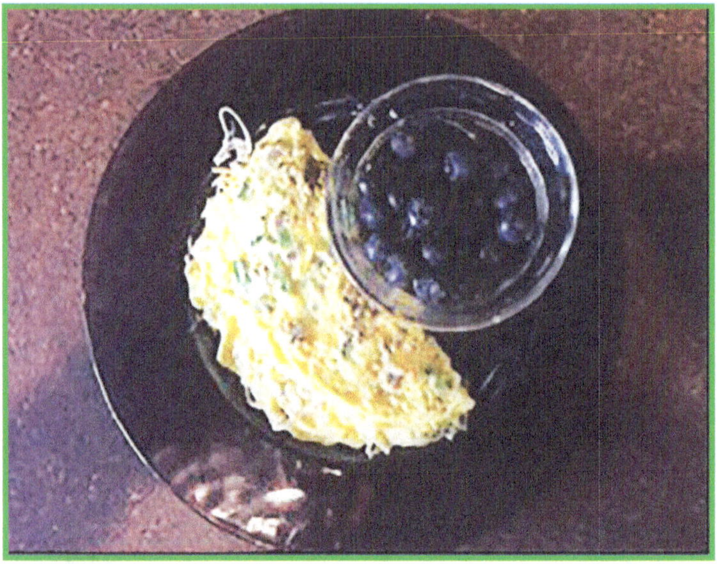

The easiest way I know to make an omelet is in a non-stick 8 inch fry pan. I drop in a bit of butter, and my ingredients, any pre-cooked meats or vegetables. When pan is sizzling I add my beaten eggs, and swirl and cook until it is firm enough to flip. Using a wide spatula, I flip the eggs, add shredded cheese and fold.

Notes

Scrambled Eggs with Ham

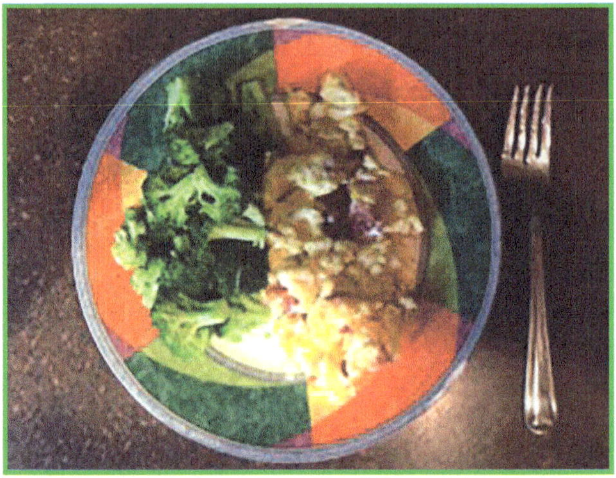

This is an easy one! No instructions necessary.
Love it with roasted broccoli from last night's dinner.
Serve with berries or grilled vegetables.

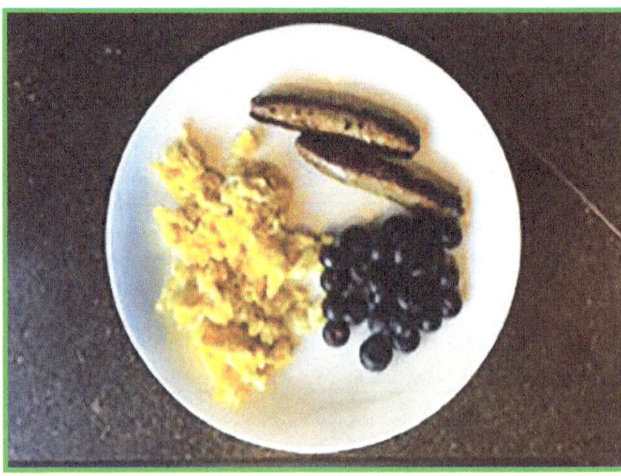

Basted Eggs

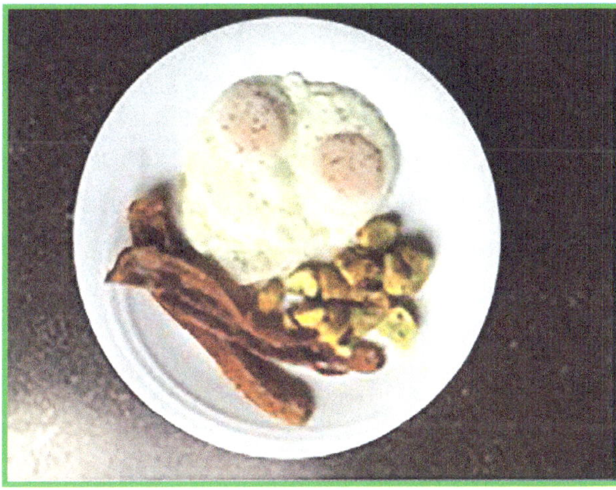

1. Heat butter, olive oil, or coconut oil in small fry pan.
2. Drop in eggs, cook till whites start to become firm and white.
3. Add a few drops of water and cover.
4. Steam to desired hardness/softness of yolk.

Serve with bacon and left over squash from dinner.

Extremely Awesome Egg Scramble

1. Sauté vegetables in butter and garlic.
2. Vegetable ideas: celery, onion, cauliflower, peppers, broccoli, mushrooms, etc.
3. Add any cooked meat ingredients if desired: Sausage, ham, bacon, etc.
4. Push vegetables & meat to the sides of the pan. Add eggs in the middle with a little salt and pepper. Scramble and mix in all ingredients.
5. Add shredded cheese if desired.

Quiche Lorraine & more…

Layer in bottom of spring-form pan or 9” pie pan for a crust-less version, or on top of almond flour pie crust.

Ingredients

2 c. shredded Swiss cheese
Finely chopped onion
Bacon bits
Whisk in bowl
4 eggs
1 c. heavy cream
1 c. almond mild
Salt & Pepper to taste
¼ tsp cayenne
Pour over cheese/onion/bacon

Variations

You can substitute cooked seafood and/or any cooked vegetables, broccoli, red peppers, mushrooms, cauliflower, asparagus, etc.

Almond Flour Pie Crust

Ingredients

2 c. almond flour (Optional: replace 1/3 cup of the almond flour with regular flour for smoother crust)
1 egg
¼ tsp. sea salt
2 tbsp. melted coconut oil

Instructions I

n a food processor, blend the flour and salt. Add egg and pulse a few times. Pour in the coconut oil slowly while running the food processor until the mixture forms big clumps or a ball.

Use this mixture as you would any pie crust dough.

Low Carb Pumpkin Pie/Bars

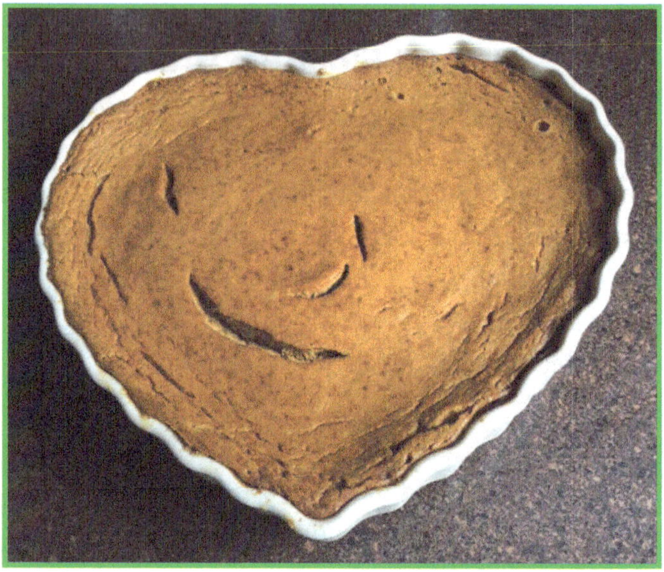

This is another winner...always a hit on holidays and parties! I just adapted the recipe on the back of the Libby's Pumpkin can, which has been a tried and true recipe since 1950. Here goes...

Ingredients

1/2 cup Splenda

1 tbsp. ground cinnamon

1/2 tsp. salt

1/2 tsp. ground ginger

1/4 tsp. ground cloves

2 large eggs

1 can (15 oz.) LIBBY'S® 100% Pure Pumpkin

6 oz. heavy cream

6 oz. unsweetened almond milk

Instructions

1. Mix Splenda, cinnamon, salt, ginger and cloves in small bowl.
2. Beat eggs in large bowl.
3. Stir in pumpkin and sugar-spice mixture. Gradually stir in cream and almond milk.

Bake in preheated 425° F oven for 15 minutes.

Reduce temperature to 350o F; bake for 40 to 50 minutes or until knife inserted near center comes out clean. Cool on wire rack for 2 hours. Serve immediately or refrigerate. Top with whipped cream before serving if desired.

Pecan Crust

Ingredients

1 c. frozen pecans
2 tbsp. melted butter
2 tbsp. almond or coconut flour

A few drops of sweetener if desired, liquid Splenda or Stevia

Instructions

1. Chop pecans in food processor, pulse till texture of small peas or lentils.
2. Add melted butter, flour, and sweetener, and press into 8" pie pan.

CHAPTER 14

Wrapping it all Up…

I recently had breakfast with a couple of my friends who struggle with their weight and are always dieting in one form or another. I realized that it seems easier for them to "go on a diet", making a shift from eating foods they are used to eating if they know it is a temporary situation. Maybe that's why going on a "diet" is a common practice and making a "lifestyle change" is less common. Why gyms are overrun with new clients in January because of New Year's resolutions and then membership wanes as people lose their inspiration and motivation. The idea of changing our lifestyle is daunting, even if it is holding us back from the life we want to live. Familiar feels safe. Limiting, but familiar.

What is it about food? What is it about our relationship with food? What is the hold it has on us? Why do some of us keep fueling our bodies with food that doesn't nourish us? What would we do if we were in a relationship with a person that was not just unfulfilling but abusive? By the same token if you had a friend that kept going back to an abuser, what advice would you offer them? What causes a person to stay in an abusive relationship; or even leave for a while and then go back?

People get used to it. Abuse feels comfortable for them, even normal. If they were in a relationship with someone who treated them with respect and dignity it would feel odd. The same goes for food. Even though eating nutritionally-vacant sugar-laden poor excuses for food makes us feel bloated and sick, we keep coming back for more. It's familiar, comforting, and we feel safe.

But take heart! The new way can become familiar, comforting, and feel safe. Ask anyone who has broken free from abuse, experienced emotional healing, and adjusted to a new way of being treated. They will never go back. And when they see a friend or even a stranger caught up in the cycle of abuse they can't help but scream out, "There's a better way!"

The new way can become familiar, comforting, and feel safe.

I hope you have seen, throughout the chapters in this book, that there is indeed a better way. I hope you understand that we were raised with inaccurate information, bad science if you will, and that if we continue eating low-fat, high-carbohydrate foods we will continue the path of increase. Increasing waistlines, diabetes, heart disease, stroke, and death. We need some insulin, but insulin resistance causes us to make too much. Eating more carbohydrates than our bodies can tolerate creates too much insulin. These factors are partly to blame for our diabetes epidemic.

Sugar-addiction is rampant in society and in order to break the cycle and become free of cravings, it is imperative that we limit our sugar/carb intake to our own personal tolerance. We can replace those carb calories with healthy fat calories, giving our bodies a long-burning fuel. If we eat LCHF, it will create keto-adaption, which means we will burn fat. Even the fat stored on our bodies!

Changing our ways requires a mindset shift. Exercise helps a lot, we feel better and we do better. It even helps our emotional health, and we can overcome emotional eating. Use the tools of social support and slogans to get into recovery. Be encouraged by Vicki's Story, a story of real-life success!

And finally...what the heck to eat, anyway? Easy guidelines for shopping, meal planning, and some tried and true low-carb recipes that the entire family can enjoy. Additional resources to boot.

Additional Reading

"The biggest reason people don't succeed is because they don't expose themselves to existing information."
Jim Rohn

There's a growing movement of scientists, researchers, reporters, doctors, nutritionists, and their patients who are blazing a path for us, into a weight normalizing and blood sugar stabilizing way of life. A yellow brick road to a healthy future. The following list is by no means a comprehensive list of all the work being done in the fields of LCHF nutrition, ketogenic diets, and exercise science. The authors are scholars whose work I admire, whom I follow online and read their books, papers, and articles. They all agree that in order to achieve good health we need to minimize excess sugar and insulin in our blood. I am grateful for their input into my own health and the health of my family, and hope you will dive in deeper and continue learning.

Books and Websites:

Michael Eades, MD and Mary Dan Eades, MD: *Protein Power "ProteinPower.com"*

Gary Taubes: *Why we Get Fat and What to Do About it*

Gary Taubes & Peter Attia: *"nusi.org"*

Peter Attia, MD: *"EatingAcademy.com"*

Ron Rosedale, MD: *"DrRosedale.com"*

Jimmy Moore: *"LivinLaVidaLowCarb.com," Keto Clarity, The Ketogenic Cookbook, Cholesterol Clarity, Fasting Clarity*

Dana Carpenter: *"HoldTheToast.com"*

Jenny Ruhl: *Blood Sugar 101*

Jeff Volek, MD and Stephen Phinney, MD: *The Art and Science of Low Carbohydrate Living, The Art and Science of Low Carbohydrate Performance, The New Atkins for a New You*

Eric Westman, MD*: A Low-Carbohydrate Ketogenic Diet Manual*

Dr. Dom D'Agostino: *"KetoNutrition.blogspot.com", "KetoNutrition.com"*

Steve Parker, MD: *The Paleobetic Diet: Defeat Diabetes and Prediabetes with Paleolithic Eating and Conquer Diabetes & Prediabetes: The Low Carb Mediterranean Diet*

Andreas Eenfeldt, MD: *"DietDoctor.com"*

Nina Teicholz: *The Big Fat Surprise*

Mark Hyman, MD: *Eat Fat, Get Thin*

ABOUT THE AUTHOR

Kim Minert, CD (Certified Diabetic) created this designation so she could have letters after her name like all of her friends. As a Type 1 diabetic she earned this credential attending daily classes in the School of Blood Sugar Management, with test scores less than 100. Who knew it would be a better grade to score 80 than 100 in any school...but in this one it is the case.

Diagnosed with Insulin Dependent Diabetes at the age of 44 was quite a shock, needless to say. Kim tackled the situation with education first, but found a lot of conflicting information both in books and on the internet. It was through obsessive observation of her own blood sugar, and careful correction from her doctor that she discovered what is really true. That truth is becoming more evident and accepted every day as science proves out what the low-fat, high carbohydrate dogma has done to our waistlines... and our health right along with it.

The journey of achieving normal blood sugar and getting off the yo-yo dieting roller-coaster has brought Kim to the point of finishing her first book and following the dream of helping others. Encouraging people to stabilize their blood sugar, achieve a healthy weight and have a steady stream of energy is her way to give back to the people who have led her in the journey so far.

This transformational journey from Eating Disorder to Diabetes to Healthy Living will inspire the world as it has her local following of friends and family. She re-defines the word "healthy" with stories of real people eating real food that produces a sense of well-being and satisfaction. That's right folks, no cravings once and for all.

CONTACT KIM

If you're looking for an engaging speaker for your organization…
If you want an interactive workshop…

If you would like a diabetic talk that is downright entertaining and at the same time beneficial and educational…

If you would like custom, personalized one-on-one coaching from someone who's been there and done it…

call Kim.

Pick up the Phone! (or email ☺)

Kim Minert
602-527-2341
kim@kimminert.com
www.kimminert.com

For information and to purchase Keto OS,
(Ketone Operating System)
A miraculous supplement that gives you all the good stuff, like
Better Sleep
Better Energy
Better Fat Burning
Better Focus
www.mynewbff.pruvitnow.com

To purchase Dr. Eric Westman's Adapt Your Life Products, Great on the Go Fuel Source

www.kimminert.com

NOTE TO SELF

I, _______________________ , have made the wise decision to burn Fat for Fuel and eliminate fattening carbohydrates, which will provide a steady stream of energy for my body and reduce hunger and cravings.

I begin today, ____________________ .

I have created a plan to follow, cleaned my pantry and refrigerator from temptations.

I am shopping and cooking and eating LCHF on a regular basis. I am making LCHF choices in restaurants.

I use slogans to effectively change thoughts that might de-rail me and send me down a negative path.

I have created a support system, which includes these friends and/or professionals to encourage me on my journey.______________________________

____

I am active and participate in regular physical activity which includes

____

____

____

Signature _________________________________

Notes

Notes

NOTES

CPSIA information can be obtained
at www.ICGtesting.com
Printed in the USA
FSOW03n1401060416
18894FS